turn back the clock without losing time

turn back the clock

# without losing time

## A Complete Guide to Quick and Easy Cosmetic Rejuvenation

Rhoda S. Narins, M.D., and Paul Jarrod Frank, M.D.

THREE RIVERS PRESS • NEW YORK

Published by Three Rivers Press, New York, New York.

Member of the Crown Publishing Group, a division of Random House, Inc.

www.randomhouse.com

THREE RIVERS PRESS and the Tugboat design are registered trademarks of Random House, Inc.

Printed in the United States of America

Design by Jan Derevjanik

Illustrations by Nicole Kaufman

Library of Congress Cataloging-in-Publication Data

Narins, Rhoda S., 1941–
    Turn back the clock without losing time : a complete guide to quick and easy cosmetic rejuvenation / by Rhoda S. Narins and Paul Jarrod Frank.
        p. cm.
Includes bibliographical references.
1. Surgery, Plastic—Popular works.   I. Frank, Paul Jarrod.   II. Title.

RD119 .N374 2002

617.9'5—dc21                                              2002018134

ISBN 0-609-80871-0

10 9 8 7 6 5 4 3 2 1

First Edition

To our loving families, who make everything
possible and share in our triumphs

## acknowledgments

We thank the following people for all their
contributions to this book: our illustrator,
Nicole Kaufman; our editors, Margot Schupf
and Annetta Hanna; and Charlotte Libov.

# contents

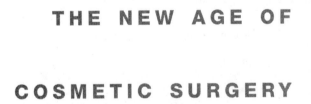

# THE NEW AGE OF

# COSMETIC SURGERY

Fifteen years ago, cosmetic surgery was reserved for celebrities and the very wealthy. These patients were mostly women who had plenty of money and lots of free time to recover. In those days, there were no options other than procedures involving lengthy hospital stays, which were followed by seclusion and elaborate cover-up stories, and cosmetic surgery was viewed as vain, at the least, and shameful at the worst!

But these are exciting times in the world of cosmetic dermatology. Now there is a far wider choice of easily accomplished treatments that don't require lengthy recuperation. There's no need for that cover-up story, because many of these treatments are done so quickly—sometimes over a lunch hour—that no one will notice. There's no more social stigma either. Indeed, it's estimated that about 2.7 million procedures to erase facial wrinkles, like peels and dermabrasions, and 300,000 liposuctions are performed annually. So it's possible some of your friends have undergone such treatments with no one but themselves the wiser. The only tip-off may be that they look rested, more youthful, or more fit or shapely, depending on what they've had done.

In *Turn Back the Clock Without Losing Time,* we introduce you to the wide array of procedures that can give you a more youthful and vital appearance without the risks of general anesthesia, invasive surgery, or the lengthy downtime that are hallmarks of the past. These treatments range from chemical peels and BOTOX, which take only minutes, to minilifts and liposuction, which can be done on an outpatient basis, without or under local anesthesia, often without the patient ever stepping into a hospital.

But there is one very important thing to remember: the secret to successful cosmetic surgery treatment is to keep in mind that the goal of these treatments is to rejuvenate, not re-create. Performed by plastic surgeons, these are invasive procedures that require hospitalization, general anesthesia, and extensive recovery. A face-lift, for instance, requires the removal of tissue, the stretching and reshaping of skin, and the cutting of bone and muscle. LILAX, on the other hand, is a far less invasive procedure that combines liposuction, laser treatment, and a small incision. It is performed by a dermatological surgeon and entails far less risk, cost, and recovery time.

All of the techniques discussed in this book will have you back on your feet either immediately or in up to four days tops—depending on what procedure you choose.

But undergoing cosmetic treatments and procedures is not the only way to look your best. For that reason, we've divided our book into three parts. In the first, What Cosmetic Treatments Can Do for You, we explore treatments and procedures that can help you turn back the clock—with a minimum of downtime.

This includes BOTOX, filling substances, peels, laser treatments, liposuction, and more.

In the second part, What You Can Do for Yourself, we'll show you which treatment or treatment combinations work best for your problem areas, such as crow's-feet, sagging redness, lines around the mouth, brown spots, reddened face, deep furrows, fat accumulations, thin lips, and more.

The final section, Putting It All Together, is a guide that will show you how the techniques and procedures combined are used to solve the most troubling problems.

So are you ready? Then without losing any time, let us show you how to turn back the clock!

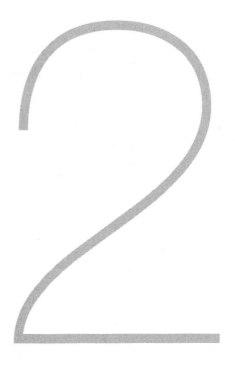

# GREAT EXPECTATIONS

There are many, many cosmetic procedures to choose from. But it's very important to make certain that those you choose are the right "fit" for you.

First you need to address some basic issues, such as asking yourself what type of change you expect.

If you are looking for a drastic change—if you want to look like someone else entirely (a runway model perhaps), look decades younger, or match the "ideal" image of what you've always wanted to look like—these procedures may not be for you. Your expectations may be so high that you would inevitably be disappointed, no matter what the outcome. Cosmetic surgery works best for those already happy with themselves but who want to improve realistically their physical appearance.

Cosmetic surgery is for self-improvement, not perfection. If your expectations are too high, you're bound to be unhappy. If your expectations are realistic, you will almost always be satisfied.

Are you doing this to look younger? It's only natural to want to look as young as you feel. Often, the way we feel about ourselves (and how others feel about us) is based on our reflection in the mirror. Face it; we live in a youth-oriented society. Happily, subtle differences in your appearance can result in dramatic changes, both in the way you view yourself and the way others view you.

There are a variety of reasons you may want to look younger. Maybe you need to compete with younger people in the job market, or you're a baby boomer and you're growing older but don't want to look it. Some of your friends may already have taken the plunge and are looking great!

Midlife changes (such as divorce), career bumps, or just plain ego can also inspire you to revamp your appearance. Tom, a fifty-five-year-old computer technician, was downsized from his job. Going from interview to interview, he couldn't shake the feeling that he was a victim of age discrimination. While it's illegal to be asked your age when you apply for a job, it's not hard for an interviewer to guess. In Tom's case, his thinning hair, paunchy physique, and full face made him look ten years older. After a hair transplant and liposuction, he soon landed a coveted job. Did his better appearance or his newfound confidence in looking his best help him? No matter; he's now happily employed.

Lila, at seventy, was retired and financially secure. An attractive woman, her lovely skin belied her years, but the excess fat and skin on her neck gave her away. Liposuction gave her a firmer, more sculptured jawline. Within a few weeks, she felt more confident and landed the library job she had sought. She also began socializing more. Some people may think that having cosmetic surgery makes you a superficial person, but as these examples demonstrate, that's not true. The truth is that we judge each other first on appearance—and sometimes that first appearance is the only chance you get.

You may wonder when you should begin having cosmetic procedures. Cosmetic procedures are *not* just for older people. That is a common misconception. Cosmetic enhancement can improve your self-esteem and rejuvenate your looks just as living a healthy lifestyle does. The earlier you start, the more gracefully you'll age. You also may require fewer major procedures later on to maintain your youthful appearance.

Consider Linda, for instance. When she came into our office, she seemed rather embarrassed. "My friends say it's silly for me to be concerned about wrinkles at my age. I'm not even thirty-five years old. But I've noticed these lines forming around my mouth and I'm upset because they make me look older already. So I thought I'd see about getting them done now, rather than later," she said.

Linda was right in her assessment. At her present age, her wrinkles are finer and not deeply etched into her face; a chemical peel will be a great help now, and with treatments every few years, she'll stave off the deep type of wrinkles that would require more strenuous treatment later.

Delores decided to wait until she was fifty-five and then have "everything" done. With her combination of wrinkles, lines, and age spots, she needed a $CO_2$ laser resurfacing, which requires downtime. She would have looked better longer if she'd come in sooner.

On the other hand, it's never too late to consider cosmetic procedures. An increasing number of techniques are ideal for

# THE AGING PROCESS

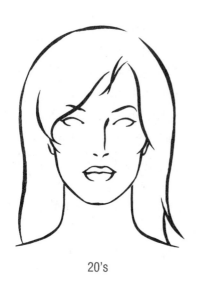

20's

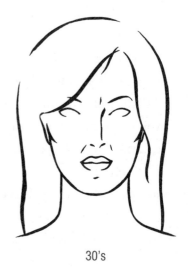

30's

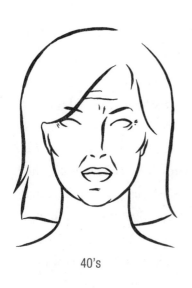

40's

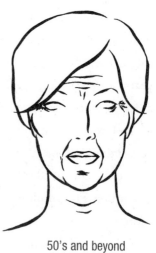

50's and beyond

older patients who don't want to subject themselves to significant recuperation time or risk.

So what should you do first? Educate yourself. Actually, you're doing that by reading this book. Also, be discerning about your sources of information. We are constantly being bombarded with information from our youth-and-beauty obsessed media. This is both a blessing and a curse. On the positive side, television news shows, magazines, and the Internet are great resources for information. The problem is that much of this information is of questionable validity. Often, the procedure presented is cast as a panacea with no discussion of the risks and, most importantly, the result that can be realistically achieved.

You can expect wonderful results from today's cosmetic procedures but not miracles. For example, microdermabrasion, which can be done as a series of lunchtime treatments, does a wonderful job of exfoliating the skin and getting rid of superficial pigment problems, acne, and areas of roughness. But it cannot get rid of wrinkles or acne scars. Other examples of media hype are creams that supposedly "lift" your face or other body parts, or machines that promise to rid your thighs of cellulite. Always be wary of sweeping claims about guaranteed results. The more that is promised, the more skeptical you should be.

Once you've thought about what you'd like to achieve through cosmetic surgery and evaluated your options, the next step is probably to find a qualified medical professional. Cosmetic surgery is very lucrative, so physicians such as internists and gynecologists, who have a different field of expertise, are increasingly performing these procedures. But just knowing how to perform these procedures is not enough. Cosmetic surgery is an art requiring specialty training and experience. Dermatologic surgeons and plastic surgeons are the best specialists for these treatments.

Why a dermatologic surgeon? *Dermatology* means that which relates to the diagnosis and diseases of the skin. However, dermatologic surgeons are skilled not only in diagnosing and treating diseases of the skin but also in providing cosmetic treatments.

Dermatologic surgeons are physicians who are trained and experienced in a wide variety of surgical and nonsurgical methods of treating the skin and preventing skin problems. A dermatologic surgeon must complete medical school, a year of internship, and at least three years of specialized residency training in the specialty. This residency includes not only treating diseases and disorders of the skin, hair, and nails, as well as developing expertise in the treatment of skin cancer, but also training in the treatment of sun-damaged skin and the cosmetic improvement of the skin. Because of this expertise, dermatologic surgeons have been referred to as the "masters of your appearance."

An appointment for a consultation with a dermatologic surgeon is a good place to start. The doctor should ask you what goals you want to achieve and draw up a treatment plan, beginning with the least extensive procedures. Often a combination of treatments will provide the physical boost you're seeking. If more extensive treatment, like a face-lift, is desired, the doctor can refer you to a plastic surgeon. While both dermatologic and plastic surgeons perform cosmetic procedures, a plastic surgeon often reconstructs tissue down to the bone and performs more invasive procedures.

Dermatologic surgeons usually specialize in procedures that remain in and above the muscles, with particular expertise in treating aging of the skin and skin care. Often this is all you will need. Because her face was networked with wrinkles from years in the sun, Selma was concerned that she needed a face-lift. It turned out, though, that skin resurfacing through a series of chemical peels was all that she needed.

Make sure the physician you select is board certified. Though you may think, Well, this is only cosmetic surgery, you should still chose your dermatologic surgeon with utmost care. Cosmetic surgery, while performed for the sake of appearance, is a medical procedure, and although the risks are few (especially with the type of less-invasive treatments we're discussing), you still want to guard against the complications that can occur.

Board certification ensures that the doctor has completed not only the formal specialized education required after medical school but also has passed examinations to attest to his or her knowledge of the selected specialty. A good dermatologic surgeon is not necessarily board certified, but if you select one who is, you are automatically assured that your doctor has at least gone beyond the minimum in acquiring training and knowledge. Read on to find the solutions that will work best for you.

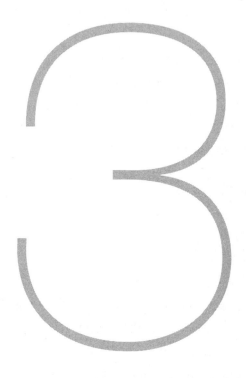

# A SKIN PRIMER

You picked up this book because you want to look your best. To do that, though, you need to understand a few basics as well as little of the biology involved.

Why? Well first, the snake-oil salesmen of the past may have vanished, but some facets of the cosmetic industry are close behind. Hundreds of skin and beauty products — no, probably thousands — are available to the consumer. Almost all these products claim to provide a younger, fresher-looking you. As you'll learn throughout this book, some of these claims are valid, but many more are hype. Once you understand a little of the biology of your skin, you can take the right steps to keep it looking its best.

Second, after reading this book, you may very well decide to seek a professional who can help you achieve the results of procedures discussed in our book. Knowing a bit about the science of skin will help you better choose and communicate with the dermatologic surgeon you select and also help you choose among the options you are presented.

Third, although we are talking about appearance, it's wise to bear in mind that skin abnormalities are not only unsightly but can also be signs of disease. Skin cancer is at epidemic proportions. Knowing a bit about this disease is not only worthwhile, it can also save your life. We'll talk more about that later on.

## your skin

The skin is not simply a fixed covering for the rest of the body; the skin also controls temperature and serves as a barrier to the outside elements.

The skin is comprised of a multitude of layers more broadly divided into three big layers: the epidermis, the dermis, and the subcutis (the fatty layer).

The epidermis is what we show to the world. The epidermis itself is made up of four different layers. The top layer of the epidermis contains the remains of dead skin cells. These dead cells are useful because they help protect the skin, but they can also make the skin appear dull. These dead cells slough off naturally, but you can also use substances, in particular alpha hydroxy acids (AHA), to cause exfoliation, or the shedding of these cells.

The epidermis also contains melanocytes. These cells contain melanin—the dark pigment that gives our skin its color. We all have the same number of melanin cells, but they vary in the amount of melanin they produce; dark-skinned people have more melanin than light-skinned people. People who tan rapidly, after being out for five minutes in the sun, have more melanosomes, which are the pigment-filled sacs that fill the melanocytes and spread out rapidly when exposed to sunlight.

The epidermis is extremely thin, and beneath the epidermis is the dermis. The dermis contains different types of cells and glands and provides durability. The dermis includes the functional glands of the skin, including the sweat glands, which produce (not surprisingly) sweat; the sebaceous glands, which produce oil; and the hair follicles, which produce hair.

The dermis is mostly made up of collagen. Collagen makes up 70 percent of the dermis and is also an ingredient in about 70 percent of the skin-care products designed to replenish it in your skin. Do these products get through the skin barrier and actually work? That's never been shown to be the case, although you couldn't tell from the claims beauty product manufacturers make in their advertising.

Your dermis also contains a substance called elastin, which is similar to collagen and so named because it gives the skin its elasticity. There is also another important substance in the dermis, hyaluronic acid, which holds in moisture.

Below the dermis is the fatty layer, the subcutis. This layer both protects and cushions. The blood vessels and nerves are contained here. Fat also plays an important role in the way our body metabolizes glucose (sugar) and hormones.

As we age, the composition of these skin layers changes. When we're babies, we have a thicker fat layer. As we grow older, we lose this "baby fat," and as adults, the dermis and the epidermis become thinner and the dermis loses its elasticity. Wrinkles, lines, and "aging skin" are the results. Restoring that youthful quality is one main goal of the procedures outlined in this book.

# marks and lesions

Numerous types of marks and lesions can appear on the skin as we grow older. It is important to know about the different types of marks and lesions because this book covers the various ways to have unsightly ones removed.

Some, like moles or nevi, are predetermined before birth; others, like freckles or solar lentigo, are caused by sun exposure. These are usually referred to by dermatologists as "lesions," which simply means a growth.

## brown lesions

These flat brown spots, formally known as solar lentigos and informally as liver spots, are caused by sun exposure. They appear in exposed areas, including the face, chest, back of the hands, arms, and legs.

## seborrheic keratoses

As you grow older, these crusty, warty brownish lesions can appear. You can develop none, one, or up to hundreds of these lesions.

## moles

Moles are known medically as nevi. These skin-colored or brown lesions can appear at any age.

## actinic keratoses

Also known as solar keratosis, these red scaly areas usually appear on the skin of light-skinned people. They are caused by sun exposure and can be precursors to skin cancer.

## chloasma

Chloasma is a brown discoloration of the face usually seen in women. The cause is hormones or birth control pills. This can be lightened with bleaching agents.

## red lesions

This condition is usually seen on fair-skinned people, often those with rosacea, a facial disease that can have many different manifestations, including dilated blood vessels, acne cysts, rosiness, scaly red patches, and conjunctivitis.

Types of red lesions are:

- Telangiectasia—dilated blood vessels within the skin that appear on the face and are particularly common on the sides of the nose.

- Cherry hemangiomas

- De Morgan angiomas—small red circular lesions that are generally hereditary and benign.

- Spider hemangiomas—small red spots with little red lines emanating from the center that blanch when you press them.

Now that you have these skin basics under your belt, you can better understand how the techniques and procedures we discuss can keep your skin looking younger, clearer, and at its best.

part 1

# What Cosmetic Treatments Can Do for You

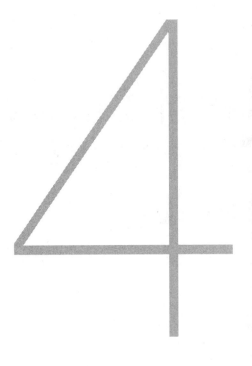

# STAY YOUNG WITH BOTOX

Valerie, an attractive woman in her late twenties, was determined not to appear old any sooner than necessary. At a young age, she had decided to undertake a skin maintenance program to keep looking good. She wore a wide-brimmed hat in the sun, used sunscreen, and refused to bake in the sun, like her friends. But she was increasingly concerned about a deepening frown line between her eyes. She mentioned this to her mother, who had the same line, only much deeper, and they came for a consultation together.

While Valerie was concerned about the line making her look prematurely old, her mother had other concerns. "Because of this frown line, people always think I'm angry or mean," said Valerie's mother, who was actually a sweet-tempered woman. Both women opted for Botox injections. Their frown lines disappeared, and they were ecstatic with the results. "This has completely changed people's perception of me. Before, they spoke to me defensively, because they thought I was angry. Now, I not only look better, but everyone is friendlier," Valerie's mother said. Wrinkles are the most common—and dismaying—signs of aging, especially the deep creases between the eyes, crow's-feet, and frown lines. Happily, BOTOX can make these obvious signs of growing older vanish, with no downtime. And the effects last for up to six months.

BOTOX is made from the bacterium that causes botulism, but its medical use now, for over a decade, is completely safe. This is because of the minuscule doses that are used and because it is used locally instead of systemically.

# erasing wrinkles

There are numerous ways BOTOX can enhance your appearance. BOTOX can get rid of the deep crease between your eyes, eradicate crow's-feet, erase the lines on your neck, smooth your skin texture, prevent new lines from forming, and even stop you from excessive sweating (hyperhidrosis). BOTOX also can eliminate "dynamic" wrinkles, which are those that appear when you change expressions, and prevent new lines from forming.

BOTOX erases wrinkles because it temporarily prevents the release of acetylcholine, an important physiologic neurotransmitter that causes muscles—including facial ones—to contract. BOTOX was introduced to dermatologists by neurologists and ophthalmologists, who used the toxin to treat uncontrollable muscle spasms of the eye and other parts of the body. They noticed that not only did the spasms cease, but their patients' wrinkles also softened.

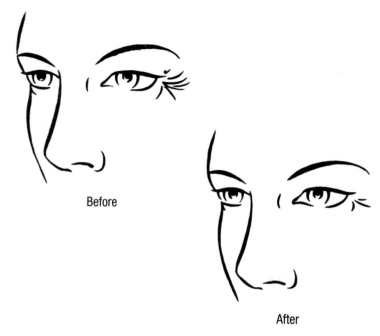

Before

After

BOTOX FOR CROW'S FEET

A major cause of wrinkles, in addition to tanning and smoking, is our natural use of facial muscles. Hundreds of years ago, aristocratic mothers would warn their daughters not to smile too much. They were right; our constant use of these muscles since birth results in the wrinkles, crow's-feet, and lines that make our faces look stern later on. With BOTOX, specific muscles are selectively relaxed, including the frontalis, which causes frown lines on the forehead, the procerous, which forms the line in the glabella area (the "frown" lines between the eyes), the orbicularis oculi, which form crow's-feet, and the platysma, which is the muscle that forms lines in the neck. BOTOX not only softens the lines but

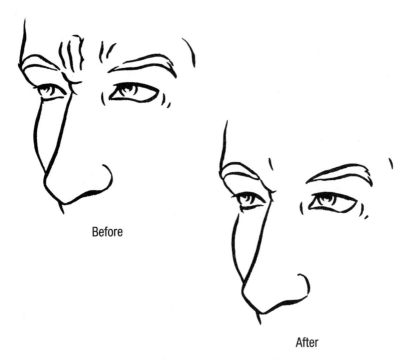

Before

After

BOTOX FOR GLABELLA FOLDS (FROWN LINES)

because the muscles are prevented from contracting, it also prevents new ones from forming. Thus, BOTOX also acts as a wrinkle preventative, making it appropriate for both young and old patients.

## the treatment

BOTOX is injected with small needles into the desired muscle group. The patient experiences a slight burning and occasionally bruising at the site. You shouldn't lie down or participate in aerobic activities for a few hours after treatment to ensure that the BOTOX remains in its designated site. But, other than that, you can resume your normal activity immediately. Anywhere from five to ten days later, just when you're convinced the BOTOX didn't work, you awaken one morning and realize your wrinkles are softer. Over the next two weeks, they will vanish. You'll also find yourself unable to contract the muscle that caused the wrinkle, but you won't miss it; you'll be able to smile and move all the facial muscles you need to. In fact, you'll realize you never needed to flex that wrinkle-causing muscle at all.

While a BOTOX treatment may sound like a breeze, you need to carefully select the doctor who performs it. There is a delicate art to administering BOTOX, and the doctor should be very experienced, with an extensive knowledge of musculature of the face. It isn't easy to paralyze certain muscles without limiting your facial expression. There are standard injection protocols that he or she will follow, but your doctor should study your facial movements carefully and treat you based not on a textbook chart but on your own specific musculature.

## taking the sweat out of being "sweaty"

Since muscles and sweat glands share the same neurotransmitter, BOTOX can be used by those who sweat excessively in their armpits, hands, and feet. Several injections right under the skin in the desired areas after topical anesthesia stuns the sweat glands for six months at a time. When used on the hand, the only side effect may be the inability to make a tight grip. But no more sweaty palms—for about six months anyway. You can stop ruining your clothes and running up your dry cleaning bills with all those terrible armpit stains. BOTOX works great in this area. This is a good option for those who are sensitive to deodorants. Consider Jerry's story. "It's normal to sweat, but not like me. Shaking hands, which I have to do a lot, being a salesman, was a nightmare for me. So were ruined shirts and suits. I tried every deodorant under the sun, but nothing worked." But that was until he tried BOTOX. "Now, no more sweats. I feel much more comfortable."

An alternative to BOTOX for treating excessive sweating is liposuction. Liposuction can be performed very superficially under the skin. With its opening aimed upward toward the undersurface of the skin, a cannula is used to scrape out some of the sweat glands. Testing is performed first to make certain this is the area that is the sweatiest. Usually this is done on a small area of about one and a half to two inches.

## frequently asked questions about botox

q: What are the benefits of BOTOX?

a: BOTOX is an ideal treatment for most areas of the face and for those vertical and horizontal lines on the neck caused by overactive muscles. It can also shape your eyebrows and given them extra lift, or add more of an arch. But BOTOX isn't appropriate for all parts of the face. Wrinkles above the

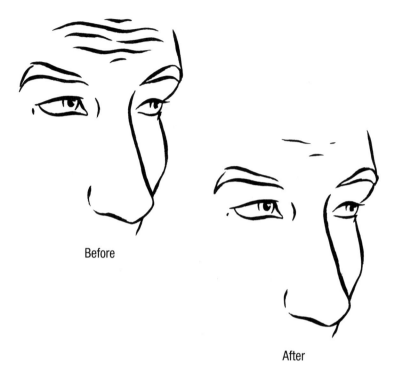

Before

After

**BOTOX FOR FOREHEAD WRINKLES**

lip and corners of the mouth are a bit more difficult to treat with BOTOX because you need to flex these muscles to talk and eat. Very low doses can be injected into these areas to get some results, but it's usually a combination of BOTOX and other treatments that work best.

q: Is there anyone who shouldn't use BOTOX?

a: BOTOX is not recommended for use above the lip or at the corners of the mouth by those who play wind instruments or who like to drink through straws. We also do not use it on women who are pregnant.

q: How long does BOTOX last?

a: The effects of BOTOX last four to six months, although all the people who love BOTOX (which is mostly everyone who uses it) contend the effect is over when it's really only 20 percent gone. They are so used to the 100 percent effect that they find any motion or wrinkle unacceptable.

q: Does BOTOX have side effects?

a: BOTOX offers one of the most dramatic changes with the least risk. Minor side effects can occur if BOTOX migrates to muscles that shouldn't be shut down. For example, when treating the glabellar complex (the crease between the eyebrows), lid lag (tired eye) might occur. This usually lasts only a few weeks and can be treated with eyedrops to stimulate the muscle until it bounces back on its own. When BOTOX is injected around the mouth, it can temporarily cause weakness of the area or a cosmetically undesirable asymmetry. If BOTOX migrates when used around the eyes then it can result in double vision and headaches; when it is injected around the neck, it can lead to trouble swallowing. Fortunately, these adverse reactions are extremely rare. Again, all of these effects, if they occur, are temporary.

Don't be a BOTOX bargain hunter. A BOTOX treatment can cost anywhere from $400 to $1,200, depending on the number of areas treated and the level of the doctor's expertise. BOTOX is an expensive and delicate agent. It comes in a vacuum-sealed frozen powder that requires reconstitution with saline, and if it is not used within twenty-four hours of this, it loses its effectiveness. If you choose a practitioner solely by price, you run the risk of getting less potent BOTOX, and your wrinkles will return sooner.

Like many other things, when it comes to cosmetic surgery, you get what you pay for. So don't hunt in a bargain basement for your beauty and health. You're worth more than that!

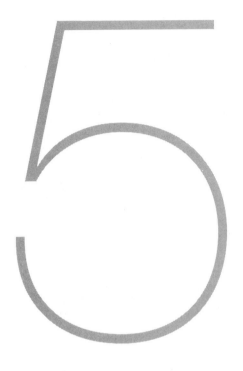

# RESURFACE YOUR SKIN

Think back to the last time you saw a crew resurfacing an old, cracked road. Didn't the resulting miles of fresh surface look great? Cosmetic resurfacing is like that. The treatments that fall under this category are some of the easiest, most effective ways to rid yourself of old, wrinkled-looking skin and reveal the smooth, firm, youthful you underneath.

There are three types of resurfacing: chemical peels, physical peels, and laser peels. Choosing the one that is right for you depends on a number of factors, including how much improvement you wish, what you want to spend, and how much recovery time you can afford.

Chemical peels use certain chemical agents, such as fruit-based and other types of acids. Physical peels, such as dermabrasion and micro-dermabrasion, are performed with abrasive instruments that sand away the old skin. Laser peels (discussed in the next chapter) are performed using high-energy light sources that target the water in skin and thermally destroy those unwanted lines. All three methods work by exfoliating unwanted tissue. Basically, the top, dull layers of the skin are removed, stimulating new skin growth and leaving a brighter, younger appearance. Depending on the methodology and the level of penetration, these procedures can also remove the wrinkles that you spent years developing.

Resurfacing is also categorized according to depth: light, light-to-medium, medium, and deep. The type and depth of the resurfacing you need depends on the condition of your skin and the results you want. Younger people, with smooth skin, may benefit from a light chemical peel, such as a glycolic peel, or microdermabrasion, a light sanding. These procedures give skin a radiant glow and can also help get rid of acne and blackheads. For those with acne, light resurfacing is an excellent way to unclog pores. Light chemical peels don't truly affect wrinkles, although they improve the texture of the skin. Those over thirty who want to deflect the signs of aging will find a medium-depth procedure more appropriate, which can produce younger, firmer skin that will last for months or even years.

Light resurfacing affects only the epidermis, which is the uppermost layer of the skin. Medium resurfacing gets down to the upper layer of the dermis—the second layer—and deep resurfacing affects the mid-to-deep layers of the dermis.

In the case of light and light-to-medium peels, the recovery period ranges from nothing to a few days of reddened skin, which isn't too much of a price to pay for the peel's freshening effects. Medium-depth procedures produce an effect similar to having a weeklong sunburn. Deep resurfacing is usually performed using a $CO_2$ laser or a chemical called phenol. These more intensive procedures carry greater risk, often require weeks of recovery, and aren't appropriate for most of us.

# chemical peels

Chemical peels are the most commonly used resurfacing agents. They are safe and people are usually delighted with the results. Depending on the agents and their concentration, peels can be superficial to deep, depending on how they penetrate the top layers of the skin. Complications can include whiteheads, infection, and cold sores. These procedures are "technician-dependent," and an experienced physician knows how to avoid such problems. If you are prone to cold sores, tell your doctor so you can be given an antiviral agent prior to the treatment. You typically will be given one anyway, but this way you can be sure.

People with fair skin usually can tolerate peels better than those with darker skin. Chemical peels (except light ones) are not to be used on those with darker skin—including African-Americans and Asians—because of the risk of discoloration. Those with darker skin are less prone to wrinkles anyway because of the protection their pigment affords their skin.

## light peel

Light peels are also called "superficial," "freshening," or "lunchtime" peels. A light peel removes the top, dead layer of the skin's cells. No sedation or local anesthetic is needed, so you can get right up and go about your business. Right after the peel,

**turn-back-the-clock tip**

A combination of treatments or peels often works best. For instance, a chemical peel can be used to make your complexion glow, while a local laser peel gets rid of those unattractive lines around the mouth. Then, a filling substance is used to make the wrinkles around the lips vanish. Voilà! The total result is a much younger looking you.

your skin may redden and flake a little, as if you've spent too long in the sun. This fades too. Within a few days, a nonvisible shedding of the skin will commence. The revealed radiant skin lasts for days—long enough for Cinderella's ball and a little bit afterward. For these peels, a variety of acids, such as 10 percent trichloroacetic acid (TCA), 70 percent alpha hydroxy, or 8 percent beta hydroxy acids, such as salicylic acid, are used.

Make sure you know which agent your dermatologist uses. If you have an adverse reaction to one, you should avoid it in the future.

One of the most popular peels is called glycolic rejuvenation. This peel is performed using glycolic acid (an alpha hydroxy acid), a natural nontoxic fruit product derived from sugarcane. By lightening age spots, fading discoloration, and temporarily improving the appearance of superficial wrinkles, it can make your skin look more youthful and feel softer. It also improves the texture of the skin. This peel is used on dark-skinned people because it usually doesn't alter skin tones.

A light chemical peel should be done in a series for the best effect. It should be done initially every three weeks, then after the first three to four weeks, the treatments can be spaced out to every four to six weeks.

turn-back-the-clock tip

Beware of "spa" peels. They are equally expensive but often less effective. Aestheticians working in spas (or elsewhere) are not allowed to use the concentrations of agents that dermatologists are licensed to use.

## light-to-medium peel

A light-to-medium peel is exactly what it sounds like—this is about halfway between a light and a medium peel. The recovery time is a little longer, but the effect also lasts longer.

A light-to-medium peel involves a variety of agents; the most commonly used is Jessner's solution, which is 14 percent each of glycolic acid, salicylic acid, and resorcinol. Another frequently used agent is low-concentration trichloroacetic acid (20 percent), which is used at higher strengths for medium-depth peels.

The light-to-medium peel has all the benefits of a light peel but is especially good for those with acne, dark spots, or general skin discoloration. The side effects, which are similar to sunburn, include reddening and peeling, and are a little more visible and last a little longer than those of a light peel. The advantage is that you can really start taking years off your skin with this type of peel. Light-to-medium peels are also ideal for treating sun damage on all areas of the body that are more sensitive than the face. Treating your arms, hands, neck, back, and the V-neck part of your chest will keep you confident every time you wear your favorite summer dresses.

## medium peel

The medium peel is a mainstay of dermatology. The process is the same as for a light peel, but a stronger chemical formula is used—usually 35 percent TCA over Jessner's solution, glycolic acid, or a similar agent. The side effects linger longer; your face will become dark red or brown for a few days, and for a week you will appear to have a bad sunburn. Your skin will peel like a bad sunburn as well.

This peel rids your face of fine lines and significantly evens out your skin tones. Deep lines won't be removed, but they will be softer. Brown marks and blackheads will vanish, and sun-damaged skin appears smooth and fresh. Actinic keratoses, which are dry scaly spots from too much sun that can turn into skin cancer, also disappear.

Once your skin finishes peeling, you will find the skin underneath looks great—not too pink or too red. Then, after several weeks, your body begins to manufacture collagen, that all-important natural protein, thereby producing firmer-looking skin. This process will continue for several more months, resulting in tighter skin. So by undergoing a medium peel once every few years, you can maintain your skin at a lovely level. Medium peels are also often done in conjunction with face-lifts, because although the face-lift tightens, it doesn't improve the surface condition of the skin.

# physical peels

Physical peels act like chemical peels, but abrasive materials instead of chemical agents are used to remove the outer layers of the skin.

Dermabrasion, a treatment to remove scars or wrinkles with instruments such as a diamond fraise, revolving wire brushes, or sandpaper, is an effective treatment, but it does require downtime. However, a new, quicker, and gentler form of dermabrasion has become popular over the past two years. This new form, microdermabrasion (also called minisanding) is relatively new and has become an extremely popular technique. Microdermabrasion softens the skin, evens out color, and leaves you looking radiant.

But, like the glycolic peel, the effect is temporary, and it doesn't remove wrinkles, despite what you may have heard.

For this procedure, very tiny crystals are used to polish the skin. As with a light peel, there's no downtime, and you can have microdermabrasion performed over a lunch hour. Again, a series of treatments is needed to achieve the best results.

As technology advances, newer, more aggressive machines are enabling doctors to penetrate deeper into the skin to achieve a greater cosmetic result. Unfortunately, we all know the old adage no pain, no gain. This means that the deeper you go, the more recovery time before your skin becomes smoother, softer, and glowing.

If you have some sensitivity to the agents in light chemical peels, microdermabrasion may be just the procedure for you. There's also a deeper procedure, called dermabrasion, in which a rotating brush or a diamond fraise is used to sand off the face. This is very good for severe acne scarring and wrinkling, but $CO_2$ laser resurfacing is now the preferred technique because it is more effective and safer. Dermabrasion is also good for deep lines. However, both of these procedures, although very effective, require at least two to three weeks of recovery time, so we won't go into them in much detail here.

## frequently asked questions about peels

q: What is the best way to have peels done?

a: For the best results, have the peels done in a series, allowing some time to pass in between. These small incremental

improvements allow you to slowly develop a more glowing appearance.

q: What is the recovery period necessary for the different
types of peels?

a: The recovery period for light and light-to-medium peels
ranges from nothing to a few days of reddened skin, which
isn't too much of a price to pay for the peel's freshening
effects. Medium-depth procedures produce an effect similar
to that of a weeklong sunburn. Unlike a sunburn, however, a chemical peel does not involve solar radiation, so it
does not damage the skin the way excess sun does. Deep
resurfacing is usually performed using a $CO_2$ laser or a
chemical called phenol. These more intensive procedures
carry greater risk, longer recovery (one week for $CO_2$
laser, two weeks for dermabrasion and phenol peels), and
aren't appropriate for the vast majority of us.

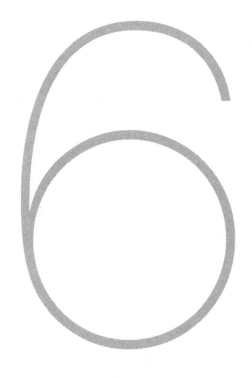

# LASERS AND YOU

Once the domain of characters like Flash Gordon, the Jetsons, and Darth Vader, lasers are now part of our everyday lives. Lasers are used in modern weaponry and medicine, and now the power of the laser has been harnessed to the service of beauty. In the hands of a dermatologic surgeon, known as a laser surgeon for this purpose, lasers remove wrinkles, scars, red spots, dark spots, rosacea, and spider veins. They also help erase tattoos, remove unwanted hair, and diminish congenital defects such as port-wine stains.

Since they have become so prevalent, patients tend to think lasers are the answer to everything. Every day in our practice, when we recite a list of options to patients, invariably one will pipe up, "But why can't a laser do that?"

Yes, lasers can do a lot, but they aren't magic. They are, however, a valuable piece of technology. In the last twenty years this technology has dramatically transformed the field of cosmetic surgery, and it is still developing at an amazing pace.

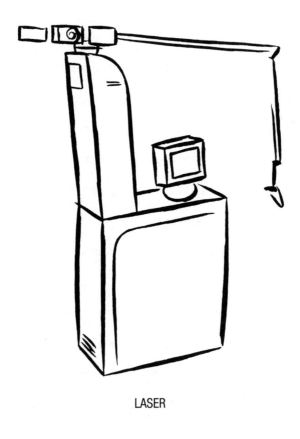

LASER

Laser is an acronym for Light Amplification by Stimulated Emission of Radiation. This means that a laser is a focused beam of light at a specific wavelength. In many ways, lasers are just very fancy knives that use thermal energy, or heat, as a means of destruction. As laser surgeons, we use these instruments to destroy, shape, or stimulate a variety of targets. This is accomplished without burning or injuring any of the surrounding tissue.

How is this possible? Imagine a square of blacktop in the middle of a grass field. After a few hours of sunshine, you'll find that the blacktop is very hot to walk on while the grass remains quite comfortable. Because the tar pigment absorbs the light, the blacktop absorbs more heat. Similarly, a laser's thermal energy is drawn to hair follicles and dark or discolored areas of skin.

There are many different kinds of lasers, and certain substances absorb certain laser wavelengths better than others do. When using laser technology for cosmetic corrections, it's necessary to choose the laser instrument that is right for a precise use. In other words, a different laser needs to be used with different targets. The targets most commonly used in laser skin surgery are water (which makes up 90 percent of the skin tissue), hemoglobin (which gives blood its red color) and melanin (the brown pigment in our skin).

For example, most red problems on the skin, whether they are spider vessels, flushed skin, or scar redness, are due to an overabundance of blood vessels in the area. We use a type of laser light that is specifically absorbed by hemoglobin, so blood in the target vessels is heated and the target vessels destroyed with little or no damage to the surrounding tissue.

You may have heard or read about machines that use "pulsed light." Unfortunately, this is one of those jack-of-all-trades devices that does a little of everything but does no one thing well. These devices claim to treat everything from pigmented and vascular lesions to hair removal and photo-facials. They're technically not lasers because they use not single, but several, differing wavelengths of light. The machine can potentially treat several different types of problems, but usually none of them well. So although these machines sound wonderful and are of some value for simple problems, they do not match the efficacy, safety, and ease of using a laser that specializes in treating a specific type of problem.

Remember that lasers cannot treat everything, and they do not always remove the entire targeted area, even when used on the particular type of problems they can treat. For instance, although in sclerotherapy lasers can be used to treat conditions such as varicose veins, another option that costs less is a much better treatment.

# skin problems

## dark spots (pigmented lesions)

Our skin gets its color from pigment. The major pigment in the human body is melanin. We see it in our skin, our hair, and our eyes.

Dark or brown spots, known also as "liver spots," "age spots," or "pigmented lesions," are one of the earliest and most noticeable signs of aging. These are often the result of sun exposure. Laser skin surgery can remove these spots. But the process is not that simple. Melanin is everywhere in the skin and absorbs, to some degree, many different wavelengths of light. So the surgeon must be careful not to destroy the wrong pigmented areas, namely, normal skin.

You may wonder why the laser doesn't also remove the normally pigmented skin. This is because the laser light selectively targets dark concentrations of melanin. If after the abnormal concentrations of melanin are removed the treatment then continued on normal skin, then some whitening could occur. However, the body's natural regenerative system would replace the normal melanin after a period of time, returning the skin to its natural state.

At least 80 percent of all common pigmented lesions are removed with one treatment. If a lesion covers a large area, the physician may want to treat the area in several stages, to avoid unnecessary discomfort.

Several different types of lasers are used to treat dark spots. The most common is the Ruby laser, which very specifically targets dark pigments including melanin and dark tattoo pigment (tattoo removal is discussed later in this chapter). This laser works best on light-skinned patients. But there are many other lasers that can be used. The Q-switched Nd:YAG, the Diode, and the Alexandrite lasers are used for the same purposes, but they have a better safety profile in darker-skinned patients.

There are also nonlaser treatments that can be done to treat dark spots. Liquid nitrogen, applied with a Q-Tip or an applicator gun, can also help lighten dark spots but may leave white spots if your skin is pigmented.

Bleaching agents can also be used. These are creams containing hydroquinone or kojic acid. Different agents can be used and sometimes combined with Retin-A. In our office, we make and use several of these combinations. After treatment the patient applies a sunblock every morning, because there's no point in bleaching any part of your skin unless you are going to prevent the sun from darkening it.

Although skin cancer can arise from moles, it's very normal to have a few dozen moles on your body, so you shouldn't think that all moles would turn into cancer. As long as there is no significant change in the size or color of a mole, it is very unlikely that the mole will ever cause a problem.

Laser surgeons are not comfortable removing moles because of the lack of 100 percent efficacy, the risk of scarring, and the potential to mask future changes in the mole that could serve as a cancer warning sign. Also, the laser cannot be used for the removal of moles that are cancerous or suspected of being cancerous. In such a case, a biopsy, the removal and examination of a small piece of tissue, must be performed. Laser treatment would render this impossible. However, laser treatment can lighten moles that are cosmetically unsightly. Moles can also be removed using other methods. For more on mole removal, see chapter 12.

## red spots (vascular lesions)

Red spots, or vascular lesions, refer to the various unsightly skin changes and conditions caused by faulty blood vessels. These include angiomas of various types. Angiomas are collections of abnormally dense vascular tissue (collections of blood vessels) usually located in and below the skin that cause red or purple discoloration. Some types of angiomas are spider angiomas (bright red areas that have slender projections resembling spider legs), port-wine stain (flat, pink, red, or purple discoloration appearing at birth), telangiectasia (enlarged vessels), and cherry hemangiomas, those cherry red bumps that occur more commonly with aging, although all ages can develop them. Other red spots and areas include overgrown or red scars (old or new), and redness or flushing commonly seen in people with rosacea. General redness associated with previous trauma and medical problems such as rosacea can also be treated, as you'll see.

These problems are treated with a laser device that destroys the blood vessels that give the skin the undesired red coloration. Consider spider veins, for instance. Unlike pigmented lesions, which can be treated successfully with several different types of lasers, these vascular lesions are clearly best treated with a type of laser referred to as the Pulsed-dye.

Originally, the Pulsed-dye laser generated a wavelength that directly destroyed the blood vessels, but this resulted in eggplant-colored bruising that lasted for up to two weeks and was difficult to cover up. Thanks to improved laser technology (the V-Beam laser), the energy can now be spread out in a fashion that minimizes or avoids this reaction. Even when bruising occurs, it should last only a few days and can be covered with makeup. Although, in most cases, the Pulsed-dye (V-Beam) laser offers the best treatment options, there are other lasers that can be used. For spider veins on the face, the Diode and HGM lasers and pulsed light machines, which use similar wavelengths of light, are used. These lasers never cause any black-and-blue marks, but they don't work as well, and the improvement is often temporary.

## rhinophyma

Laser treatments can help treat a special problem called rhinophyma. This is a reddish thickening of the nose that is the result of chronic rosacea, a common skin condition that causes redness of the forehead, cheeks, and nose. Over time, this can give the nose a larger, irregular size and warty configuration. In cartoons, it has been portrayed as a "drunk's nose," but this occurs from rosacea, not from drinking (although alcohol use, eating spicy foods, or anything that causes flushing can aggravate the condition). Laser resurfacing of the nose with a $CO_2$ or Erbium YAG laser can peel off skin and reshape and decrease its size. The major downtime is several days of redness, but this treatment can make a dramatic difference. Treatment with the V–Beam laser can remove the redness. This requires less down time and is often enough to make an appreciable difference.

# frequently asked questions about laser treatment of skin problems

q: How many laser treatments are needed?

a: The number of treatments needed depends on the size, location, depth, and color of the blemish. Some vascular discoloration, such as facial spider veins, may require only one treatment. In the case of facial redness and flushing, one to three treatments are usually needed. If multiple treatments are needed, they should be spaced about a month apart. This will allow time for proper healing. During this time, the redness becomes progressively lighter.

q: Is laser treatment painful?

a: Most people who have experienced this type of laser treatment describe it as a minor discomfort rather than being painful. The actual laser pulse is so short that, like other types of laser treatments, it feels more like a rubber band snapping on the skin. An initial warm, stinging sensation quickly subsides after each pulse. Most adults tolerate this slightly uncomfortable sensation without the need for anesthetics. But if children are being treated for a congenital blemish, for instance, an anesthetic may be required.

# hair removal

It's ironic; we all want more hair in some places and less in others. Traditionally, the main ways to remove unwanted hair were by using chemical depilatories, waxing, tweezing, or electrolysis, which removes unwanted hair with a needle using an electrical current inserted into the hair follicle. Some methods are painful, some are messy, and all are only temporary. But laser treatments can now provide a means of permanent hair removal.

Developed less than a decade ago, this procedure is designed to target the pigment (melanin) in the hair shaft, permanently damaging the follicle itself so hair doesn't grow back. Dermatologic surgeons discovered this use for laser technology while treating brown spots and tattoos. They noticed that hair that had been in the treated areas was not growing back. So, they figured, why not use the lasers to treat just hair? Well, there may come a day when there is no more need to wax, pluck, or rip, but right now, although laser hair removal is effective, there are limitations.

Not everyone has equal success using the laser for hair removal. As noted earlier, the lasers detect pigment, so, in the case of hair, the darker it is, and the lighter the skin, the better the result. Treating darker-skinned people or individuals with thin blond hair is more difficult, although lasers are recently able to treat such patients. But the good news is that, over the past two years, different lasers have been invented, enabling the removal of hair colors that were impossible before. This is particularly true of blond shades; the only colors impossible to remove now are the "white" blonds and gray.

## frequently asked questions about laser hair removal

q: What types of hair can lasers remove?

a: Lasers can help eliminate hair from just about anywhere on the body. For women, the most popular areas for hair removal are the face, underarms, legs, and the bikini area. For men, the areas are the ears, hands, knuckles, back, and chest.

q: How effective is laser hair removal?

a: The answer to this question lies in the more accurate (and FDA-approved) term for laser hair removal, which is "laser hair reduction." This means that the density of the hair can be significantly and permanently reduced with a series of treatments. In our experience, we've generally found that 70 percent of hairs can be destroyed with three treatments. That isn't to say that a 100 percent reduction is impossible, but we cannot make this guarantee because, on certain patients, we may see only a 50 to 60 percent reduction in certain areas after a series of treatments. With maintenance treatments a higher percentage of follicles can usually be destroyed. A 50 to 60 percent permanent reduction is very significant!

q: What types of lasers are best?

a: Several different types of lasers can be used for hair reduction, many with equal results. Advances in the laser have had less to do with their efficacy and more to do with their speed and their ability to treat darker skin types. For example, people with dark Mediterranean skin often struggle with unwanted hair growth. However, laser treatment risked damage to their normal skin. But most people can now be treated, thanks to the use of different wavelengths, skin-cooling devices, and altering pulse width, which refers to the time in which energy is distributed.

q: How long does laser hair removal treatment take?

a: The treatment is fairly quick. Laser hair removal on the back once took up to two hours. Many of the newer lasers now go at such a fast pace that it takes twenty to forty-five minutes. This treatment is for men who in the past would have done nothing about their hairy backs, given the stigma of waxing or electrolysis.

Treatments are done in a series, spaced four to six weeks apart. This takes advantage of the hair-growing cycle to target the growing hairs, not those that are resting or degenerating. At least three treatments are required to get most of the hairs in the growing cycle.

q: What does laser hair removal feel like?

a: You will feel a mild discomfort, like the snapping of a small rubber band against your scalp.

q: What are the side effects?

a: Hives and redness can occur in the treated areas for a short time, but this only indicates the treatment worked. Unwanted side effects include blistering, changes in pigmentation, which usually returns in time, and in extremely rare cases, permanent marks. Because of the protective cooling devices now used, this procedure has become significantly less painful as well. For women, if you've had a bikini wax, this is a piece of cake by comparison. Many women say they can barely feel it.

q: What can I do if I'm not a candidate for laser hair removal?

a: If you are not a candidate for laser hair removal, there is another option. Consider trying Vaniqua, a topical cream that slows hair growth. Vaniqua, available by prescription, is for people who want to remove light blond or gray hair from their body, or for the light peach fuzz or thin wisps of hair above the lips or on the cheek. Vaniqua doesn't cause the hair to fall out, but it does slow its growth. So, for instance, if you typically have your arms waxed to remove hair every month, by applying Vaniqua daily, you could reduce the waxing sessions to once every three months. The drawback is the expense. A month's supply of Vaniqua costs about $40, and you'd have to keep up the treatment to keep off the hair. So if you're a candidate for laser hair removal, it may be more effective to have a series of from one to three laser treatments. Vaniqua may be useful, though, for the light peach fuzz or wisps of hair on the cheek.

## wrinkles and scars

The solutions to some of dermatology's toughest problems have come about thanks to innovations over the years such as laser resurfacing. Until recently, people with wrinkles from severe sun damage and scarring from acne or chicken pox didn't have options with minimal recovery time.

Laser resurfacing is a procedure specifically designed to remove superficial and moderately deep wrinkles of the face. These wrinkles primarily include those on the upper lip, crow's-feet around the eyes, and shallow wrinkles on the cheeks and forehead. Laser resurfacing is also an effective treatment for moderately depressed broad scars, such as those from acne.

Despite what the media has said about other treatments for wrinkles and scars, there was no effective treatment until the carbon dioxide ($CO_2$) resurfacing laser was developed. This is a great procedure, but it requires seven to eight days to recover after a treatment for wrinkles and eight to twelve days for acne scarring. There is also the risk of scarring, pigment abnormalities, and prolonged periods of redness, although an experienced laser surgeon can minimize these problems.

A few years ago, a less invasive laser—the Erbium: YAG—was developed. The Erbium laser offers a shorter recovery time, but it doesn't work as well as the $CO_2$ laser.

But then came a new generation of lasers. While $CO_2$ laser resurfacing still remains the leader in terms of making a real difference in treating acne scars and severe wrinkling while also treating brown marks and sallow color, more options now exist. Though laser tightening treatments achieve just 35 to 40 percent of the $CO_2$ laser's effectiveness, their advantage is that you can go out to dinner the night of the treatment.

The difference between resurfacing the skin and tightening and toning without resurfacing lies in the understanding of the term "resurfacing." True resurfacing connotes the ablation, or removal, of the top layer of superficial skin, while non-resurfacing, or non-ablative, lasers do not. The $CO_2$ and Erbium lasers are true resurfacing lasers. The other lasers resurface, tighten, and tone the skin without the removal of that skin layer. Therefore, the downtime and the risk is less, but, unfortunately, so is the efficacy.

As with most other inventions, this new technology was discovered serendipitously. After being treated with Pulsed-dye vascular lasers (the type used for this procedure) for other problems, patients noticed a reduction in wrinkles and improvement in acne scarring.

Newer types of laser skin treatment include lasers that do photo-facials, which remove brown spots and lighten vessels, dermal tightening, nonablative resurfacing, and laser toning. These are all different names given to the same procedure in which skin tightening and scar improvement is achieved using one of several lasers that do not remove the top layer of skin ("non-ablative").

First, the top layer of skin is targeted to remove the extra fold of skin that causes the wrinkle, leaving a normal skin surface behind. Second, the laser helps to correct facial wrinkles and scars by directly affecting the collagen within the dermis, the middle layer of the skin. The heat generated by the laser allows the collagen to reform, resulting in a tightening of the skin, which provides a more uniform, smooth appearance.

The beauty of laser tightening comes from the result of subtly damaging the underlying portion of the skin with thermal energy while protecting the upper layer. In this way, the production of healthy new collagen, the most abundant protein in our skin, is stimulated. The work is done from underneath, so no damage is seen from the outside because the outside layers of skin are unharmed. Lasers used for this treatment include the Pulsed-dye lasers (such as the V-Beam), the Q-switched Nd: YAG, the Cool Touch, and the pulsed light sources.

# frequently asked questions about laser skin resurfacing

q: Which laser works best?

a: What we've found in working with all of these lasers is that there is no best choice for everything—all require a series of treatments. All work to some degree. All are done with no downtime. Good results involve using a combination of different lasers with different wavelengths of light. This is another reason to go to a laser surgeon who is an expert.

q: How long are the treatments and how many are necessary?

a: Depending on the extent and type of laser used, the procedure may last anywhere from several minutes to one hour. Patients generally experience mild to no discomfort after treatment.

As with many cosmetic treatments, patience is required. To get the best effect, usually at least three to six treatments are needed, separated by two to six weeks. Since the skin is regenerating from the formation of new collagen that starts in three months, it takes three to six months to notice an improvement.

q: How effective is laser skin tightening?

a: Full-face procedures with overall tightening provide the best result. This is because doing laser resurfacing of any kind on the entire face results in uniform skin tones instead of a "patchy" effect.

Also, the most satisfied patients are also those who are realistic. Beware of advertising that oversells these techniques. These treatments don't erase wrinkles and scars, but they do soften them. Lines, wrinkles, and scars don't disappear completely, but they become less noticeable.

As with most things in life . . . no pain, no gain. For drastic changes, measures more drastic than laser tightening are usually necessary. The $CO_2$ laser resurfacing procedure may be what you need. Still, these laser skin tightening treatments appear to be the wave of the future.

# tattoo removal

Although it does not usually fall into the category of cosmetic treatments, tattoo removal can be very important to a person's appearance. The tattoo that was a terrific idea in the 1960s, 1970s, and 1980s and beyond may now be marring your appearance. Alas, it's much easier to get a tattoo than to remove it.

Tattoos are pigmented lesions, so the lighter the patient's skin, the easier the tattoo is to remove. Also, tattoos are basically implanted foreign bodies, so it's easier to remove tattoos put on by amateurs than those that are professionally done. On the average, professional tattoos require five to seven treatments, while amateur tattoos require three to four treatments, all spaced approximately one to two months apart. The number of treatments depends on the amount and type of ink used and the depth of the ink in the skin. Usually, fewer than ten treatments are needed.

Different laser devices must be used, depending on the color ink in the tattoo. This is because the wavelength of the laser light used varies, depending on the color. Black tattoos on white skin usually can be completely removed without much risk. On the other end of the spectrum, an Asian person seeking to remove a multicolored tattoo can expect a variable degree of fading with a greater chance of some scarring and pigment alteration. Many people, though, prefer a faded version to the original tattoo.

Dark (blue/black) inks and red inks fade the best, and oranges and purples usually respond well. Green and yellow inks are the most difficult to remove, although additional treatments can produce significant fading. Unfortunately, even though technological improvements are making it easier to remove different colors, tattoo artists keep coming up with new, more elaborate designs and colors that are difficult to remove.

Bear in mind that over 100 tattoo inks are in worldwide use today, none of which are regulated by the FDA. Not knowing which tattoo ink was used, how deep it was injected, or the amount used makes it impossible for a physician to predict how successful any given tattoo removal will be.

Tattoo removal is generally not any more painful than any other laser skin surgery treatments. The impact of the energy from the powerful pulse of light is similar to the snap of a thin rubber band or specks of hot cooking oil on the skin. Most patients do not require anesthesia.

Usually there will be pinpoint bleeding associated with the treatment. An antibacterial ointment and a dressing are applied to the area. The patient will also probably be given an ointment to be applied at home. A shower can be taken the next day, although the treated area should not be scrubbed.

Laser tattoo removal usually costs several thousand dollars, depending on the size, the colors, and the patient's skin type.

To summarize, when it comes to removing tattoos, lasers are not magic wands. But they are significantly better than several of the more invasive and scarring techniques that were used before.

**turn-back-the-clock tip**

If you consult a laser surgeon about the removal of a multicolored tattoo, make sure he or she has several different types of lasers available. Unfortunately, today's technology does not offer one machine that treats all colors effectively.

# frequently asked questions about laser skin surgery

q: Who is the best candidate for laser skin surgery?

a: The ideal candidate for laser skin surgery is generally light-skinned. This is because laser wavelengths do not differentiate well between dark spots and dark skin tissue, so on a darker-skinned patient, they can target the normal skin as well. This doesn't mean that if you have darker skin you are automatically not a candidate for laser skin surgery, but it means that the laser surgeon must be extra cautious. Blistering and scarring can occur. Also, darker-skinned people may experience a temporary increase (or decrease) in pigmentation postoperatively. Fortunately, this alteration in pigmentation is usually temporary.

Thanks to progress in this area, more options are becoming available for those who are darker skinned. With the newer technology for treating red lesions, such as the V-Beam (candela laser), which we prefer, and the V-Star (cynosure laser), we can protect the normal skin with a coolant spray or jet of air. This allows us to be more aggressive with difficult lesions and to minimize some of the complications associated with darker skin tones.

As with other cosmetic surgery, it's important that a skilled laser surgeon evaluate your type of problem, its severity, and, most importantly, your skin type, before deciding which procedures to use. Also, how your skin will react and the side effects you'll experience can usually be predicted beforehand, depending again on your skin type and the type of problem you are having treated.

q: How much do laser treatments cost?

a: The cost of laser treatments always varies, depending on the type and extent of the lesion. But generally each treatment can run between $300 and $700. Some problems can be dealt with in a single treatment, but in many cases, a series of treatments is necessary. So depending on the size and complexity of the problem, the cost can run from several hundred to several thousand dollars.

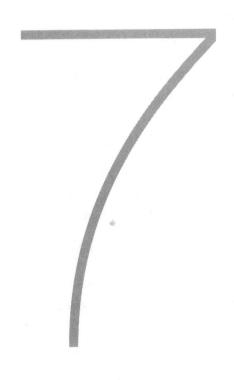

# 7

**FILLING IN YOUR FLAWS**

You may think wrinkles are the most obvious effects of aging, but try this: look at your face in the mirror, and then compare what you see with a picture of your face from years ago. See what we mean? It isn't just the lines that give away your age, although, of course, they are there. It is also the depressions and hollows of your face that make you look older.

Fortunately, there is a way to remedy these signs of aging. With the use of filling substances, such as collagen, Dermalogen, or implants of your own soft tissue, your face can be smoother, less drawn, and younger looking. These are among the most important products and techniques available for cosmetic rejuvenation.

As we age, the bony structure and fat distribution in our face dramatically change. These changes occur below the surface of our skin. We can't see them happening, but we certainly have to live with the result.

Similar changes are also occurring in the rest of our body. As we grow older, proteins and natural sugars such as collagen, hyaluronic acid, and elastic fibers are markedly reduced in quantity and quality.

Fortunately, dermatologic surgeons have helped develop several ways to combat these changes by actually returning or redistributing these substances back to the skin. We can accomplish this at several levels—either superficially or deeper. Sometimes a combination of treatments is needed.

For instance, as our patient Sandra aged, she found herself bothered by the increased hollowing of her cheeks, which she thought gave her a skeletal look. Her physician chose to use fat implants to give her cheeks a more pleasing, rounded shape and collagen to erase the vertical lines above her lips.

Using filling substances to augment soft tissue offers exciting opportunities for enhancing your appearance. It can achieve effects ranging from subtle to dramatic, because you can limit or increase the amount of material injected. So you can tailor the change you want to suit the look you want, or what your pocketbook dictates.

There is one drawback with some of these filling substances; they do not create permanent changes. The exceptions are fat transfer, which in some cases may last very long, if not forever, and silicone. However, temporary results are not necessarily a drawback, because if you aren't pleased with the results (although most people are), you don't have to live with them forever.

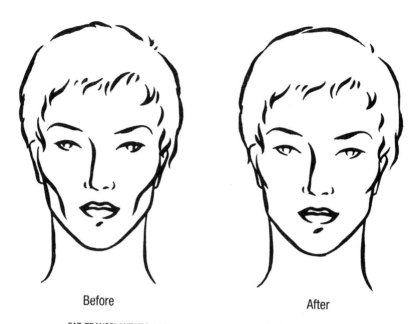

| Before | After |

FAT TRANSPLANTATION FOR HOLLOWED CHEEKS AND FACIAL CONTOURING

Here's a rundown on the most important of the multitude of filling agents available to treat the aging face.

## filling agents

### collagen

Collagen makes up much of the human dermis and is among the most abundant proteins in our bodies. So when seeking a soft tissue filler to make large wrinkles and lines vanish, it was only natural to turn to collagen, and indeed, it has become the most popular substance for this use. The collagen is injected into tar-

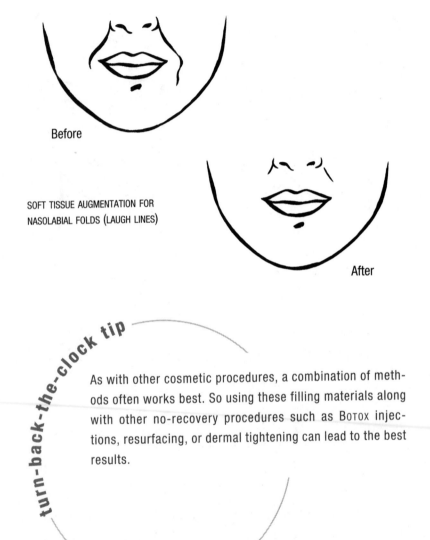

Before

SOFT TISSUE AUGMENTATION FOR
NASOLABIAL FOLDS (LAUGH LINES)

After

**turn-back-the-clock tip**

As with other cosmetic procedures, a combination of methods often works best. So using these filling materials along with other no-recovery procedures such as Botox injections, resurfacing, or dermal tightening can lead to the best results.

get wrinkles using a tiny needle and syringe, where it restores fullness and firmness to the skin. More than 1 million people have safely received collagen injections since 1977. The most commonly used form of collagen is bovine collagen, obtained from the skin of American cows raised for this purpose in a closed herd. Just in case you were wondering, no cases of animal or human disease have ever been documented in any country from using this substance. We believe that both the screening and the processing involved to develop the agent significantly limit the possibility of such an occurrence.

Bovine collagen is available in three forms: Zyderm I, Zyderm II, and Zyplast. Injecting Zyderm I and II superficially gets rid of etched-in lines and scars. Zyderm II is thicker than Zyderm I and can be used in areas where the skin is not thin. Zyplast, the third and most concentrated form of collagen, is injected deeper to fill out folds and hollows. Zyderm is often layered over Zyplast to completely treat an area.

The effects of collagen are immediately apparent. After having one side treated, you can look in the mirror and see an astonishing difference. The treated side will appear much younger and softer than the other side.

Collagen is successfully used on the lines at the sides of the mouth (nasolabial lines), frown lines, forehead lines, crow's-feet, the hollows under the eyes, vertical lines above and below the lips, puppet lines (the lines at the corners below the mouth), and acne scars.

Collagen is also used to get those full, pouty lips that are so popular today. As we age, our lips get smaller, so enhancing the lips gives a more pleasing and youthful look, as well as gets rid of most vertical lip lines.

Collagen results are not permanent. The injected collagen is absorbed by the body, which does not, unfortunately, replace it. A collagen treatment lasts for about five to six months for patients in their thirties to fifties, and four to five months for patients who are in their sixties, seventies, or older. Collagen treatment in the lips lasts about three months because the mouth is an area where there is a great deal of movement.

How long the collagen lasts also depends on how many treatments are done and whether the patient has had other cosmetic procedures. If you've had a face-lift or laser resurfacing or tightening, you will need less collagen replacement. Also, many patients choose a more subtle effect, so they may require repeat treatments that use less substance but more often.

The main advantages of this agent are its track record, its safety profile, and the fact that a local anesthetic is included along with the collagen. As the collagen is injected, the area becomes numb, which makes you more comfortable and enhances your doctor's ability to sculpt and rejuvenate. In addition, we use a topical anesthetic cream prior to treatment.

The few disadvantages are related to the fact that the collagen comes from a nonhuman animal source, resulting in the small chance of an allergic reaction. This happens very rarely, in only 3 to 5 percent of patients. To avoid this, the skin is tested twice during a period of six weeks before the treatment is done. One treatment provides full correction. The chance of developing an allergy after double testing is rare and occurs in only one out of every ten thousand cases. So you must undergo the allergy test to ensure this won't happen. Also, the thickness of the substance sometimes leaves bumps under the skin which can be felt, but not seen.

Collagen injections can cost anywhere from $250 to $500 per syringe, depending on the site, and usually involve one to three syringes. The quality of the results is dependent on the skill of the technician, so make sure you use an experienced cosmetic dermatologist.

## dermalogen

Dermalogen, a form of collagen that is used less often than bovine collagen, is human collagen made from tissue obtained from human tissue banks. The indications for this implant are the same as those for collagen. Patients who are allergic to collagen or who are opposed to using animal-based products may prefer Dermalogen. Because virtually no allergies to Dermalogen exist, you can also be treated immediately; no prior skin testing needs to be done.

Dermalogen is injected just like collagen, but it usually takes three monthly treatments to build up the desired area. However, some dermalogic surgeons find Dermalogen lasts longer than collagen.

# restylane and hylaform (hyaluronic acid)

We have in our bodies a naturally occurring sugar polysaccharide called hyaluronic acid. The natural effect of this substance is to retain water and elasticity in the skin and thus keep skin looking young. Unfortunately, as we age this substance also markedly decreases. But with Restylane and Hylaform, which are synthetic agents based on this sugar, there's a way to replace it.

Originally used by orthopedic surgeons to lubricate and functionally enhance damaged joints, hyaluronic acid–based agents are quickly becoming some of the premier filler agents in the market.

These two agents are the most common filling substances used in countries outside the United States, and they are awaiting FDA approval here. Restylane is a hyaluronic acid that is a thick gel made synthetically. This is a distinct benefit because there is no risk from disease. Hylaform is a hyaluronic acid made from roosters' coxcombs. Because hyaluronic acid is almost exactly the same compound whether it comes from an animal, a human, or is laboratory made, there is only an extremely small chance that it will cause an allergy. Therefore, no allergy testing is required. Treatment can be given immediately with immediate results. This is an ideal treatment for patients who are allergic to collagen because these agents can be used to treat the same areas. Furthermore, these agents, particularly Restylane, are reported to last longer than collagen. Unlike collagen, these substances cannot be given with built-in anesthesia, but most people don't need it. The debate is going on as to whether Restylane or Hylaform is better. Although Restylane appears to be better due to the nonanimal source, there are reports that it may have a higher chance of producing a skin reaction. Which substance lasts longer is also yet to be determined. The FDA is currently comparing the longevity of Restylane to that of collagen at six centers, including ours.

## silicone

Once a popular filling substance, silicone was used in hundreds of thousands of patients with terrific results. But although it was considered a great filling agent for years, it was never FDA approved for this use. However, it had the advantage of being a permanent filler that could be used for several different types and depths of skin defects. Unfortunately, people using impure products, overzealous use of silicone, and bad publicity related to silicone implants have squelched its use over recent years. But silicone may be coming back. The FDA has approved a newer, purer type of silicone for use in the eye to reattach retinas. Studies are planned for the use of silicone as a skin filler for the treatment of wrinkles.

Although not FDA approved as a filling substance, silicone is sometimes used for this purpose in a microdroplet technique as an off-label use, which means that it is approved for other uses but not specifically for this one. This is not that unusual a practice; for example, BOTOX is narrowly FDA approved for ophthalmological use but is now a mainstay of cosmetic dermatology and should be approved for this soon.

Silicone is useful in all the areas where collagen is used, including nasolabial folds, crow's-feet, forehead and frown lines, lip augmentation, puppet lines, and acne scars. It can also be used for cheekbone and chin augmentation and, like fat transplantation, which will be discussed later in this chapter, in treating cheek hollows. Silicone is permanent and can be used to fill in any type of defect. If you don't like it, you can't remove it, but most patients are satisfied with their results.

Since silicone is an inert, nonreactive substance, no allergy testing has to be done. There is a small chance of a nonallergic inflammatory-type reaction, a lump in the skin usually when large amounts are injected at one treatment session. Anesthetic blocks usually need to be injected locally prior to using this type of implant.

## gore-tex

Gore-Tex is a nonbiologic agent made of expanded polytetrafluoroethylene, a synthetic polymer used for hernia repair and skeletal augmentation. This is true also of Softform, a type of Gore-Tex. These substances are not injected but are inserted as tiny tubes under the skin. Gore-Tex is useful in filling in very deep folds and especially in nasolabial folds in men. Once implanted, your own tissue grows around it, and this fixes the filler in place.

Gore-Tex offers permanent filling with the option to remove it surgically at any time. Large amounts of anesthesia both locally and in blocks must be injected prior to implantation, and a few days of bruising and swelling are common after the procedure. Women generally have thin skin and can feel the implant, particularly when it is used in their lips or in the folds at the sides of their mouth. Although Gore-Tex is used extensively in lips, we feel many other filling substances give better results without the need for invasive surgery and without the side effects.

# other filling agents

There are a variety of artificial and natural filling substances that are used around the world. Many are not available in the United States or are rarely used because of their side effects or their inconvenience. They are not very good agents, in our opinion, and no FDA trials are planned. There are still other techniques we have not included because they require surgery and considerable recovery time. But we are certain the future will bring an even wider choice of filling substances, including nonbiologic, bioengineered collagen, a wide use of hyaluronic acid products, the return of silicone, and the continual refinement of fat transplantation.

But although these agents may be developed in the future, there are many filling substances available right now that offer you wonderful cosmetic improvement with minimal downtime so "even your best friend won't know" why you look relaxed and younger—unless, of course, you tell her.

*turn-back-the-clock tip*

We've said it before regarding other procedures and we will say it again. Do not hunt for bargains when shopping for fillers. These are very technique-dependent procedures. In the right hands, a single $500 syringe treatment will go further than a bargain treatment for $300, because if it turns out you need two or three additional treatments, you'll be paying double or triple the price.

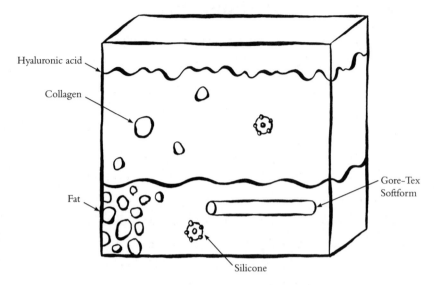

Hyaluronic acid
Collagen
Fat
Gore-Tex Softform
Silicone

PLACEMENT OF FILLING SUBSTANCES

# fat transplantation

As we age, our own superficial fat—the fat in our skin—becomes thinner. Wouldn't it be great if we could replace that thinning fat with still more fat of our own? After all, most of us have at least some we can happily get rid of, and shifting it someplace where it would look good seems to be an ideal solution. This can be done, thanks to a procedure known as fat transplantation (also known as fat augmentation or fat transfer).

The reason for the success of this procedure is that it turns out our own fat is wonderful for augmenting soft tissue in areas that need it. For better or worse, our deep layers of fat tissue do not get thinner. So, yes, we are stuck with that fat, but the good news is that it makes us our own best fat donors.

Fat can also be removed during liposuction and frozen. It will then be available for transplantation for up to two years. Only a local anesthetic is used to harvest the fat, which is reinjected immediately; the remaining fat is frozen for later use. First, a very thin cannula and syringe, along with a local anesthetic, are used to painlessly extract fat tissue from your own thigh or abdomen. Then this tissue is injected into an area where it's needed—for example, the folds or lines at the side of the mouth, marionette (or "puppet") lines below the lips, and the lines between the eyes. Also, cheekbones, chins, and lips can be built up.

Fat transplantation is not used only for cosmetic enhancement; it is also used to repair some acne scars, as well as defects after disease, injury, or surgery, and some congenital defects as well.

For instance, Barbara was very upset about a scar in an area that had sunken in on her cheek from an injury she sustained in an accident. Using just local anesthesia, Barbara's skin was separated from the muscle, then her own fat injected to lift the depressed area. Now her cheek is round and perfect, and she is thrilled with the result.

## hands

It's hard not to overestimate the importance of our hands; we constantly use them when gesturing, touching, or picking up objects. We get manicures because we're concerned about our nails, but the appearance of the hands depends on much more than just the nails.

After all, the hands take a lot of rough treatment. Our hands become calloused and marked by sun damage (too often we forget to put sunscreen on the back of our hands), and as we grow older, the skin grows thinner.

The face is not the only place where fat is used for reshaping; this is an effective technique for hands as well. Take June, for instance. She had just turned fifty and was sitting at the theater next to her daughter. Turning the pages of the theater program, she caught sight of her hands. The view shocked her! Next to her daughter's hands, June's hands looked like the hands of the middle-aged woman she is. Her hands showed her age, even though her face did not. She came in for a consultation and decided on a combination treatment. She had her hands treated with the YAG laser to get rid of the brown spots (see chapter 6), and some of her own fat was added to plump them up, ridding her hands of the skeletal, veiny appearance that had so shocked her in the theater. After the treatments, the appearance of her hands matched her youthful face.

So fat implants can be used to attractively plump up hands (an area where, unlike others, you want a little plumpness) and rejuvenate them if they've become aged and skeletal. Depressions where fat has been destroyed due to injury, disease, or surgery can also be improved.

# frequently asked questions about fat transplantation

**q:** What are the benefits of fat transplantation?

**a:** There are several benefits to fat transplantation, which uses your own body material:

- Large amounts of fat are usually available. (Finally a good use for the stuff!)

- There's no possibility of allergy, so the procedure can be done immediately and without risk of a reaction.

- Many patients get permanent results, although this varies from person to person.

**q:** How long do fat transplants last?

**a:** The length of the effect depends on your doctor's expertise in harvesting, purifying, and injecting the fat, as well as your body's individual response to it. In most patients, anywhere from 50 to 80 percent of the fat will last permanently, which gives most a lasting correction.

**q:** What is the best manner to have fat transplantation done?

**a:** Treatments should be spaced six weeks apart to give the treatment the best chance of achieving permanence. Anesthetic blocks should be used so the procedure is painless. This is similar to the type of anesthetic used at the dentist's office.

Lest we forget, for those of you fortunate enough not to have fat to spare . . . you're out of luck; you can't use other people's fat!

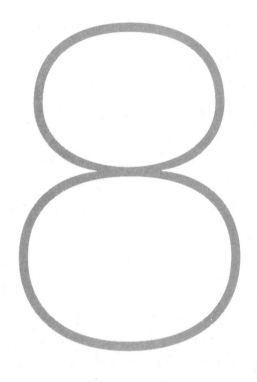

# LIPOSUCTION IN THE

# NEW MILLENNIUM

After giving birth to twins, Jennifer's weight began to climb. But it wasn't the extra pounds—it was where they were situated. Jennifer had always been proud of her flat abdomen, but now it was pouchy. In fact, wailed Jennifer, "It's a belly!" And no matter how much she exercised or dieted, the belly just wouldn't disappear.

One day she ran into her old friend Karen, whom she hadn't seen since they both graduated from college. Jennifer was stunned; Karen looked as slender as she had when they were in school. Jennifer asked Karen what kind of diet she followed, but Karen just shook her head, grinned, and said she'd undergone liposuction about a year earlier.

Jennifer was surprised. She hadn't considered liposuction. "I remember many years ago, all my mother's friends were having it done. They ended up still looking kind of lumpy, and I'd heard since that it was dangerous," Jennifer said.

"Well, that was then but this is now." Karen explained to Jennifer that this wasn't the old-fashioned kind of liposuction; this was a different type, called tumescent liposuction, that got far better results, was safe, and required virtually no downtime.

"Sign me up!" Jennifer said, laughing.

About a month later, Jennifer underwent the procedure and was delighted with the results. Instantly, most of her "belly" was gone, and as her physician told her it would, the rest vanished within the next six months. "I look like I used to," Jennifer said happily. In fact, she added, "I look better," because the new eating habits and exercise plan she'd been following since the birth of her twins had paid off.

Have you ever wished your body was a statue and the sculptor could move about it, smoothing a bit here, carving off a bit there, and contouring your body into a more pleasing silhouette?

That's nearly a description of the art of liposuction today. This is not your mother's liposuction. When the technique of liposuction was first devised, it represented a great advance over removing fat with scar-causing surgery. But the technique has advanced so much that today's results seem truly remarkable. In fact, you can just take a few days off from work and return without that protruding tummy, matronly neck, or ballooning hips.

With this kind of success, it's no wonder that liposuction is now the most commonly performed cosmetic surgery, with about 600,000 procedures performed annually. Liposuction is also among the safest of cosmetic procedures.

# what is liposuction?

Simply stated, liposuction is the removal of fat through tiny incisions in the skin using long, slim tubes called cannulas that are attached to a power suction machine. By using blunt tubes that push nerves and blood vessels out of the way but easily move through fat, liposuction was a vast improvement over the previous scar-causing fat-reduction surgery. Still, traditional liposuction was still far from ideal. Traditional liposuction, which Dr. Narins learned from the doctors who developed the procedure, still required general anesthesia, which entailed risks such as blood clots and weeks of recovery.

## tumescent liposuction

Tumescent liposuction was developed by a dermatological surgeon in the mid-1980s as a way of performing the procedure without general anesthesia. This new method greatly reduced potential complications (such as blood clots), eliminated the need for hospitalization, and shortened downtime from weeks to a few days. In addition, the anesthetic fluid used provides long-lasting anesthesia and minimizes bleeding so that there is no need for transfusions and virtually no pain.

The key to tumescent liposuction is the use of local, not general, anesthesia. This means the patient walks into the operating room and walks out afterward. In addition to all the other benefits, patients are conscious and comfortable, so they can comply with the surgeon's instructions to adjust their bodies and move into the exact position necessary to best remove the fat. This makes the surgeon's work easier, which translates into better results.

"Tumescent" refers to the type of local anesthetic that makes all this possible. *Tumescent* means "to swell." The procedure is so called because the surgeon "fills" and "swells" the fatty areas with a special numbing solution before removing the fat. With tumescent liposuction, the surgeon also uses smaller, more delicate instruments and can actually "sculpt" the contours of the body to improve your figure, rather than just remove hunks of fat.

But the innovations keep coming. New methods are making tumescent liposuction even better. The first of these was ultrasonic liposuction, and now we have power liposuction.

A surgeon performs tumescent liposuction by manually moving a cannula. But with ultrasonic liposuction, the surgeon inserts a cannula that releases ultrasonic waves into the fatty tissue to break it up before suctioning it away. Power liposuction (also called power-assisted liposuction) uses mechanical cannulas to whisk away fat instead of just suctioning it. This "electric toothbrush" type of liposuction may offer some advantages to patients and doctor. These techniques are used in conjunction with manual tumescent liposuction when necessary to get to harder-to-remove firmer areas and improve results.

## when liposuction is needed

Liposuction can solve the stubborn genetic figure problems that diet and exercise cannot. Many people work as hard as they can to get in shape but are still plagued by stubborn "problem" areas, like large hips, a protruding abdomen, or jelly roll thighs. Liposuction provides the answer to the age-old complaint about fat accumulating in certain parts of our body and why, even if we manage to lose it, the weight comes right back to the same genetic places.

The answer lies in the biology of our fat cells, coupled with heredity. The number of fat cells we have is "fixed" after puberty unless we gain large amounts of weight. Overeating enlarges these ever-present cells. Although they can be shrunk with a low-calorie diet and exercise, they still exist. That's how you gain and lose those bulges of fat associated with being overweight. Some areas have more fat cells and are more apt to enlarge after overeating. Often concentrated in the hips, buttocks, and thighs (the "violin" shape often found in women), these fat cells are stubbornly resistant to otherwise effective slimming techniques.

Heredity also plays a role in the development of these "problem areas." Chances are if your parents had them, you will too. "Like mother, like daughter" doesn't extend only to personality traits; it can extend the hips too! The beauty of liposuction is that it permanently removes some of those stubborn fat cells and gives you a smoother contour when you've long given up hope. Several generations of one family often undergo liposuction.

## uses for liposuction

In women, the areas most commonly targeted for liposuction are the neck, the arms, fat bulges in front and in back of the bra area, abdomen, hips, buttocks, waist, thighs, knees, calves, and ankles.

Women who have excess fat removed around the waist go down one or more dress sizes. Some women have excess fat in their hips, which makes wearing skirts and pants a nightmare, knees that prevent them from comfortably wearing short skirts, and calves that make them balk at sliding into fashionable boots.

## as a preventative

As with other forms of cosmetic surgery, you don't have to wait to take action with liposuction. If your mother had meaty arms, and you see yours headed that way, you can have the fat cells removed through tumescent liposuction and prevent the problem from developing further.

## not for weight loss

Liposuction is meant for body contouring, not general weight loss. Although the idea of immediately losing a lot of excess weight through liposuction seems appealing—*very appealing*—liposuction does not bring about weight loss and is not meant for the seriously obese.

One of the benefits of liposuction is that patients are often so delighted with the results that they successfully renew their diet and exercise efforts. But this change in lifestyle is just a happy by-product of the procedure.

The best results occur in healthy men and women who are thin or up to twenty-five pounds over their ideal weight. Someone who is very overweight will not recover as quickly.

Also, removing the fat through liposuction leaves unattractive excess skin that must be surgically removed later. However, there are exceptions, depending on where the fat is distributed. An overweight patient may have areas of excess fat that can easily be removed with very localized liposuction and be quite happy with the results.

## cellulite

More noticeable in overweight people, cellulite is hereditary and usually occurs in women around the hips, buttocks, and thighs. The fat in cellulite is in little fibrous packets attached to the skin. In the overweight, these packets bulge and pull the skin down in puckers. Endermologie, or suction massage, which is performed by aestheticians, reportedly breaks up the fibrous enclosures, thereby diminishing the appearance of cellulite. Liposuction is not a treatment for cellulite, but it can minimize its appearance by decreasing the amount of fat in the packets and disrupting some of the fibrous tissue bundles.

# candidates for liposuction

Mostly everyone who wants liposuction is a good candidate. Liposuction can safely be done on people of almost every age, ranging from sixteen to eighty. The best candidate is the patient of normal weight with unsightly deposits of adipose (fatty) tissue.

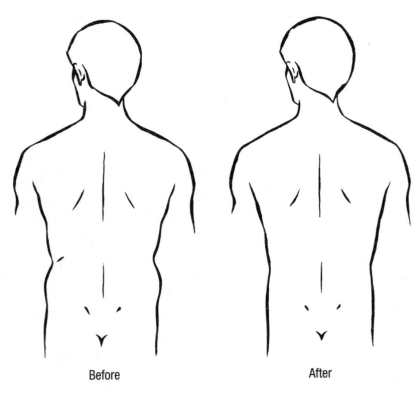

Before                                    After

TUMESCENT LIPOSUCTION OF THE WAISTLINE (LOVE HANDLES)

The patient should be in good general health (no severe heart, kidney, or liver disorders), and not be too thin: if you pinch the area targeted for liposuction between your fingers, there should be a minimum of one inch of excess fat. However, even very slender people can benefit from liposuction on specific areas. You can be very thin and still have bulges on the outer thighs, for instance.

## not for women only

Liposuction is not for women only! Just ask Gary. Except for the bulges of fat above his hipbones, Gary, forty-nine, had a fine physique. He worked out, took pride in his appearance, and looked ten years younger than his age—except for those "blasted love handles," he said. "I don't want to look like one of those middle-aged men." Gary learned about tumescent liposuction from his sister, who'd recently had her hips done. He reluctantly made an appointment, telling us, "I just don't want my friends to find out—I'd never hear the end of it." Gary underwent the procedure and was so delighted with the results that now, he says, "I can't help it. I keep telling all my friends about it. They think I look great and so do I."

Men are finding liposuction is the route to the younger-looking better build they want. In our practice, we rarely used to see a man. Now, 15 percent of our liposuction patients are men. They're tired of looking in the mirror and staring back at their father's jowls, or they don't find the term "love handles" any more endearing than do their wives. Also, many men with gynecomastia (enlarged male breasts) are very grateful to have their breasts reduced to a normal "male" size.

## expected results

Liposuction truly has changed the lives of many patients, but it doesn't work miracles. If your bodily problem comes from being big boned, liposuction won't change your body structure. But often the problem stems not from bone structure but from the excess fat covering those bones, which can be taken care of with liposuction.

You also have to keep your expectations realistic. Remember the movie *10*? Some patients are happy to advance from a "4" to a "7," while others who are already an "8" can realistically expect to become a "10." But a "7" can look darn good!

# an area-by-area guide

## face

The jowls and the cheeks above the lines at the sides of the mouth can be diminished by using very fine cannulas. This can also be done when necessary for fat at the sides of the face. Fat transfer can be done at the same time to give a higher cheekbone and fill in sunken cheeks, mandibles, nasolabial folds, marionette or puppet lines, and the hollows under the eyes.

## double chin (neck and chin)

Nothing ages a person more than excess weight in the lower face and neck, which is commonly known as a double chin. This unattractive shape makes women look matronly and gives men unwanted jowls. What is commonly known as a double chin can be easily eliminated by liposuction performed using a tiny incision in the crease under the neck and one under each ear.

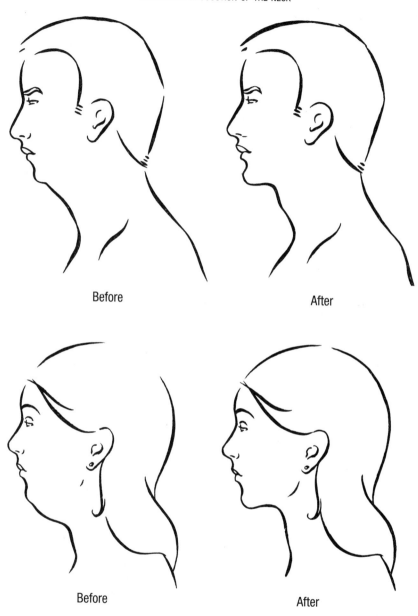

Before                    After

Before                    After

LILAX PROCEDURE

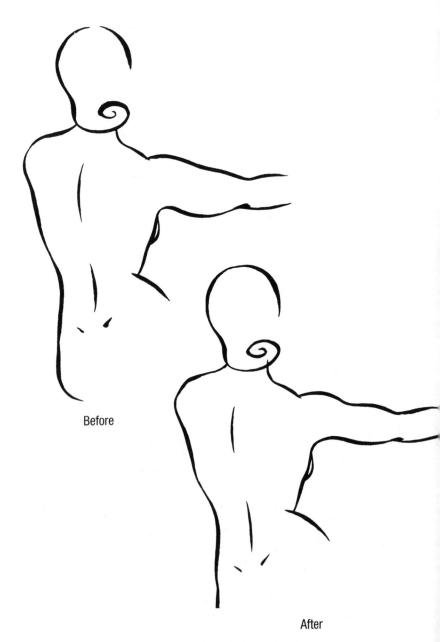

Before

After

TUMESCENT LIPOSUCTION OF THE ARMS

# pseudo face-lift: lilax

Is your problem more severe? Do you have a "turkey neck" with folds of excess skin as well as fat? This problem commonly occurs in people over sixty who are very thin. In the past, a face-lift was the only solution. But that is a drastic procedure and requires plenty of recovery time. Thanks to a combination procedure known as LILAX, you can get many of the benefits without going to all that trouble.

LILAX is a three-pronged approach: liposuction, laser, and excision. Liposuction is performed to remove fat around the neck; laser resurfacing under the skin tightens it; and a small piece of skin under the chin is excised in its natural crease so the loose skin can be lifted a bit. The result is not as dramatic as a face-lift, but LILAX is done under local anesthesia and requires only three days of downtime, which is far less than the more extensive demands of a face-lift. There is only a small scar in the natural crease under the chin. So this may be all you want—or need—to do.

Some people develop a so called dowager's hump of fat behind the neck. Liposuction can treat this as well. A few tiny incisions are used, and most can be placed where they aren't visible. The next day you can return to work or your other regular activities wearing just a binder over the area.

## arms

Sally was lifting weights in her exercise class when she looked at her arms and saw them flapping. At first she didn't even think it was her arm; it looked like her mother's arm. Her mother, alas, wasn't in the class. Later that afternoon, she had another unwelcome experience. She was trying on evening gowns for a special night and fell in love with a strapless navy blue number. "I looked at my arms and suddenly, that dress didn't seem very attractive," Sally told her friends sadly. A friend told Sally that she had just undergone tumescent liposuction in that area and was delighted with the results. Sally decided to follow suit. The day after she had the procedure, she was back at work. The only legacy from the liposuction was a tiny incision that is not visible because it was placed in the creases above her elbow. Oh, and her shapelier arms, of course. Sally bought the dress, wore it, bared her all (or at least her arms), and felt terrific.

Accumulating excess fat in your arms can give you that unflattering bulky look, a disaster when you want to bare your arms at the beach or slide into a little strapless dress after nightfall. With tumescent liposuction, excess fat is removed from the entire upper arm. This allows the skin to tighten, leaving your arms firmer and slimmer.

## chest and underarm bulges

An embarrassing problem for men is excess fat in their chest area that resembles female breasts. This can make men and boys too self-conscious to wear tight shirts or bare their chests at the beach or health club. Excess fat bulges in front and just underneath the underarms at the sides of the breast can be removed in both men and women for a firmer, trimmer look.

## "tummies" and "pots"

Most men and women despise having a protruding abdomen, known as a "tummy" or "pot." Some women notice that they

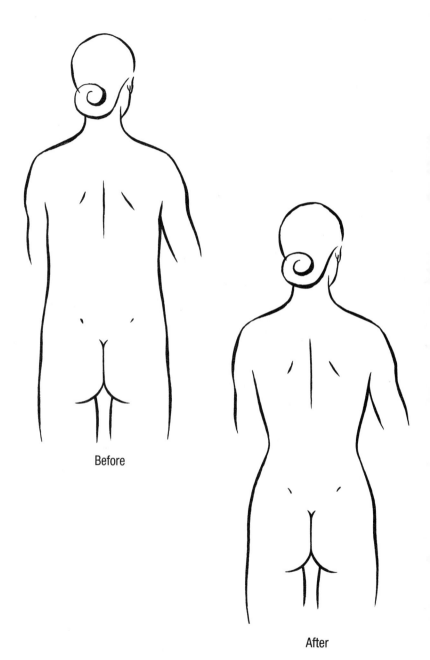

Before

After

TUMESCENT LIPOSUCTION OF THE WAISTLINE (HOURGLASS ABDOMEN PROCEDURE)

can't seem to lose their "stomach" after childbirth, or their middle expands at menopause. One solution is the "tummy tuck," but that is a more extensive procedure (but necessary if the muscle becomes loose). But liposuction alone can achieve great results in most people, without the hospitalization, general anesthesia, ten-to-twenty-inch telltale scar, and considerable expense and recovery that a tummy tuck involves.

## waistline

Not uncommonly, a woman between the ages of forty-five to fifty-five can "lose her waist" to excess fat deposits. Performing liposuction in this area can help you find that lost waistline again. Later in this chapter we'll discuss the Hourglass Abdomen procedure, which adjusts the abdomen, waist, hips, and back to create a shapely three-dimensional result.

## hips

It's no longer the 1960s; do you really want to look like a "hippie"? No, especially if you decide to slide on a pair of studded retro bell-bottoms. Some women just have large hips that make them look square and need larger clothing. This is an area that is very easy to treat with liposuction.

A combination of large hips with large outer thighs and buttocks is called a violin deformity, and the results with liposuction are really gratifying. This is an inherited trait, and the name means that, when seen from the rear, your figure is violin shaped.

"It's really hard to buy pants for a size twelve bottom when you wear a size six on top," Susan complained as she sat in our office for her consultation. Furthermore, her mother and sisters have the same big bottom and apparently her grandmother, now deceased, also had it. This was a family trait that Susan was sick of!

When Susan came in for her consultation, her mother came along. The two women had heard about tumescent liposuction from one of the mother's friends. The entire female side of the family ended up having liposuction done. Like Susan, they were delighted.

A violin deformity can be corrected easily with liposuction. And if your daughter is also taking on this shape, liposuction can be performed on patients as young as the teens.

After liposuction, that genetic shape is gone and replaced by a new, straight you. Some patients have very marked deformities, but some of our most grateful patients are those with minimal contour changes who now can really expect to be perfect.

## outer thighs

The unflattering description "saddlebags" is all too familiar to many women. This is the name given to the excess fat that accumulates on the outer thighs, because it gives the illusion of wearing riding breeches. Women with this problem may spend countless hours at the gym but find it is all for naught, because trimming this area often can only be accomplished through liposuction. You can even be extremely slim and have fat deposits in this area.

Liposuction of the upper thighs is often combined with that of the hips and buttocks to achieve the best results. Liposuction

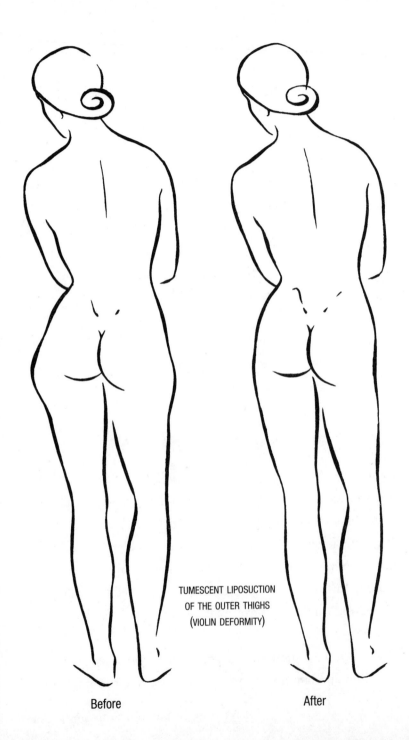

TUMESCENT LIPOSUCTION
OF THE OUTER THIGHS
(VIOLIN DEFORMITY)

Before

After

can also be performed around the thigh to reduce the diameter of the leg—a debulking procedure.

## inner thighs

The outer thigh is not the only problem area for women. Excess weight that accumulates between inner thighs can cause them to uncomfortably rub together. To solve this problem, liposuction is performed through the use of two to three incisions—one in the front of the groin, one in the buttock, and occasionally one in the back of the inner thigh.

## knees

Sometimes people think they have ugly knees because of the underlying bone structure, when actually liposuction can remove excess fat and give them slimmer knees that look good in skirts. To accomplish this procedure, one incision is generally made, and not only the inner knee can be done but also the fat pockets right on top of the knee. In addition, we always do a little bit of the upper inner calf to give the area a nice curve.

## buttocks

Some women who perceive they have "saddlebags" actually have excess fat in their buttocks. In this case, liposuction alone can be used to create a far more flattering bottom. In women with large buttocks, debulking this area can change their entire shape, enabling them to look thinner and wear smaller clothes.

## calves and ankles: piano legs

Another unflattering name for a correctable condition is "piano legs," which describes people who have excess fat around the calf and ankle. With liposuction, the fat is removed around the entire leg, again debulking it. Very small tubes are used in this procedure. Unfortunately, a few patients have big legs that are all muscle. Although you can improve the shape, you cannot debulk muscle. But for most women, the result is attractive calves and ankles.

## combos bring great results— the hourglass abdomen

In the days before tumescent liposuction, when general anesthesia was used, the operation was so cumbersome that surgeons used to try to do as many areas as possible, leading to risks and complications. With tumescent liposuction, it's easier and safer to do other areas separately. But the Hourglass Abdomen, developed by Dr. Narins, is a highly successful combination that is safe and offers striking results.

Just removing the fat from the abdomen often doesn't translate into an attractive figure. In fact, sometimes if you remove fat in the tummy but leave it at the waist and hips, you may look bulkier. The Hourglass Abdomen procedure removes excess fat from the abdomen, waist, back, and hips to create an instantly shapelier, well, shape. If you're a bit overweight, you'll end up more curvaceous. But if you're at your ideal weight, you very well may end up with a shape that's fabulous.

# frequently asked questions about liposuction

q: What is recovering from liposuction like?

a: Back in the old days, when general anesthesia was used, it sometimes took patients weeks to recover from liposuction. Now one can go back to work a day or two later and, basically, not miss a beat. There's virtually no pain, although you might feel a little sore. If you have a large buttock area that has been reduced and you have to sit, you will be sore. But 99 percent of our patients need to take nothing for pain other than Extra Strength Tylenol afterward.

If you've had a neck liposuction done—even the combination LILAX procedure—all that is required is a dressing around the neck for two or three days. Liposuction done on other parts of the body takes only a few days to recover from as well. Underneath your regular clothing you can wear a leotard, bathing suit, or just a garment with Lycra to provide extra firmness, or light support stockings if you've had a leg procedure. You can resume all of your regular activities, with the exception of jarring exercise or contact sports. But, otherwise, you can do everything you normally would, including walking, lifting weights, and using exercise bicycles and StairMasters.

q: What complications can occur?

a: Every surgical procedure carries a risk, but the ones involved in tumescent liposuction are very few.

Complications most often can occur if liposuction is performed along with more extensive procedures, such as a tummy tuck. If it is properly performed, the only complications likely to occur with tumescent liposuction are very minor ones. These include soreness, which can be alleviated by taking Tylenol, temporary numbness, sensitivity at the procedure site, bruising, and itching. Small scars that may occur at the site of the cannula insertion usually disappear within four to twelve months

q: How will I look afterward?

a: Although it's true that the final result of liposuction is best seen at six months, everyone looks better immediately. The belief that swelling occurs and makes you look worse for a while is a myth!

Sometimes a tiny touch-up may be needed post-operatively. This judgment is made four to six months afterward, and any touch-up procedure is generally short and simple.

q: Who should do my liposuction?

a: Although liposuction is considered a very safe procedure, selecting the right surgeon is extremely important. After all, the results will affect not only your health, but you'll also be looking in the mirror at them every day. The best place to start is by contacting the American Society for Dermatologic Surgery (see the Resources section). You can also ask your dermatologist or a friend who has undergone liposuction for a recommendation. Don't hesitate to travel out of town if you believe a doctor is right for you. Most experts in liposuction, like Dr. Narins, who has done over six thousand liposuction procedures, can make arrangements with hotels and transportation to accommodate patients who don't live in the area. Then schedule a consultation with the surgeon and make sure you get the answers to these important questions:

- What are the surgeon's academic credentials?

- How much experience does the surgeon have with tumescent liposuction? Make sure the surgeon uses tumescent liposuction. Remember, your surgeon should not use old-style general or intravenous (IV) anesthesia.

- Is the surgeon experienced in the ancillary techniques of power liposuction and ultrasound liposuction?

- Are patient references available?

- Are before-and-after pictures available?

- Is the surgeon conservative in his or her approach regarding how much fat can be removed at once? Although complications are very rare, you don't want a surgeon to remove too much fat at once or work on too many areas at once.

- Is the surgeon realistic about what liposuction can do for you?

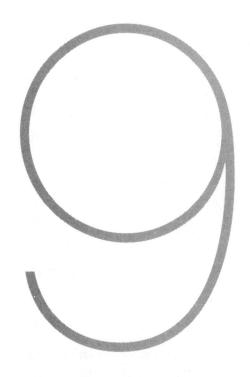

# THE "EYES" HAVE IT

"You know, I saw Patricia last week. She must have been on vacation. She looks wonderful. So rested," remarked one of our patients to us. We nodded sagely but said nothing. We know Patricia, and we knew she wasn't on vacation. She was in our office a few weeks before, having her eyelids done.

When someone looks at your face, it's your eyes that draw their immediate attention. Indeed, your eyes are said to be the windows of your soul. That's true. So if the window shades around your eyes— your lids—droop and sag, or if they are ringed with dark circles, your eyes will say more about you than you want them to. Basically, they'll say that you're old and tired-looking, when, in fact, you might feel young and energetic.

In the world of cosmetic surgery, "eye jobs" are old news. But the revolutionary news is that there are now much easier ways of solving "aging" eye problems with a minimum—or even no—downtime.

# pack those bags:
# eyelid procedures

Nothing makes you look tired and older than baggy, loose eyelids. The problem is usually due to heredity. Sometimes it can occur in people in their twenties, or even their teens.

To correct this problem, a type of eyelid surgery called blepharoplasty is performed. This procedure, discussed shortly, is excellent—when you need it. But this surgery can often be put off thanks to BOTOX and resurfacing with lasers or peels. These are procedures that can leave you looking rested and refreshed with little, or no, downtime.

## botox

The use of BOTOX has revolutionized eyelid surgery. Before BOTOX, blepharoplasty, or eyelid surgery, was the only alternative. But now, dermatologic surgeons are using BOTOX, the wrinkle-relaxing treatment described in chapter 4, to give the eyes a more wide-awake appearance. More refined techniques make BOTOX an excellent agent for reducing the number of fine wrinkles around the eyes and nose. Crow's-feet, the angry-looking "frown" lines between the eyes, and the "bunny" or "crunch" wrinkles on the sides and top of the nose can now all be treated with BOTOX. In addition, BOTOX is not only corrective, it's also preventative. It decreases the patient's ability to frown or squint, which prevents the worsening of these lines over time.

In addition, if you do opt for blepharoplasty, BOTOX can be

used beforehand to enhance the results. Afterward, the continued use of BOTOX prevents these lines from coming back.

## resurfacing

Laser or peel resurfacing can be used along with BOTOX treatments to further enhance the result. When the top layer of dull dead cells is removed fresher and firmer skin is revealed underneath. In addition, this stimulates the formation of collagen for better-looking skin. The downtime from laser resurfacing ranges from none at all to up to seven days, depending on the type of treatment selected. Resurfacing with the $CO_2$ laser takes five to seven days; a medium TCA peel takes four to six days; and the Cool Touch laser requires no downtime at all. Read more on laser resurfacing in chapter 6. Peels are explained in chapter 5.

## blepharoplasty

Also referred to as an "eye lift," or "eyelid repair," or "having your eyes done," blepharoplasty is the primary surgical procedure for erasing the eyelid wrinkles and sagging "bags" under the eye. They can be done on the lower or upper lids, or both.

As you age, pockets of fat are extruded from your eye's orbit that collect under the skin and give you a "sagging" look. These are the types of circles that look worse after you've been lying flat, eating salty food, or lack sleep. These circles should not be confused with thickened muscle, which can be treated with BOTOX.

Blepharoplasty is a procedure in which incisions are made in the natural creases or folds of the eyelids. Loose skin and extra fat

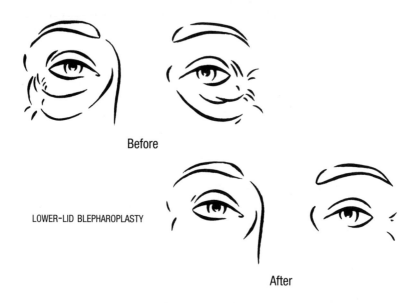

Before

LOWER-LID BLEPHAROPLASTY

After

tissue are removed. Traditionally, blepharoplasty was performed by making incisions going from the outside of the eyelid in, removing the fat, and then closing the skin, using fine sutures. It requires intravenous anesthesia and an overnight stay in a hospital. Sometimes this traditional procedure is required. But more recently a procedure known as transconjunctival blepharoplasty was devised. This procedure is performed from the inside of the eyelid out. Originally done using an electric needle, this method has again been refined so that it can be done with laser surgery. It requires no stitches and is done under local anesthesia on an outpatient basis.

Using a laser, the physician makes an incision inside the lower eyelid, where the fatty deposit is removed, leaving no visible mark. The use of the laser coagulates the blood as it cuts, which keeps bleeding minimal.

During recovery time, which takes a few days, you apply ice to your eye. Bleeding happens rarely, but you must take care not to bend over, cough, or strain while making a bowel movement. A small black-and-blue mark may occur, but this discoloration is easily hidden with makeup or sunglasses.

This wonderful procedure can make you look years younger and usually doesn't have to be repeated.

Bags under the eyes are often not the only concern; drooping upper lids can make you look older than your years as well. This is caused by an excess fold of skin or extra fat in the upper eyelid, under the eyebrow, or toward the nose.

To solve this problem, the dermatologic surgeon makes an incision along the crease in the eyelid, peels back the skin, and sculpts the underlying tissue to remove the fat pad. The pad is

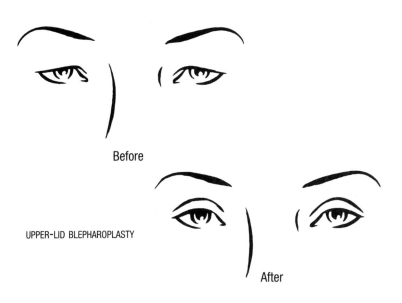

Before

UPPER-LID BLEPHAROPLASTY

After

then cauterized (heat sealed). Loose skin is removed from the exterior, if necessary, and the incision is sutured.

The postoperative effects are minimal and temporary. Stitches are usually removed after five days. Minor swelling, bruising, and discomfort should disappear within two weeks. Cold compresses will help prevent swelling.

As with other procedures, combinations can provide excellent results. So after the blepharoplasty procedures, resurfacing can be done on the upper lid or both lids.

Blepharoplasty can also be combined with BOTOX for ideal results. Blepharoplasty can rid your eyelids of extra fat and skin, but it does nothing for wrinkles. In fact, when the fat pad is removed, this can still leave a wrinkled area behind. Think of a balloon—once it's deflated, you're still left with a wrinkled piece of plastic. In this sense, BOTOX is a way of tightening that outer skin around your eye and removing the wrinkles.

The result of blepharoplasty? Your lids won't feel as heavy, it will be easier to put on makeup, and you won't look so tired. As with Patricia, friends will marvel at how rested and refreshed you look.

## the brow lift

In addition to sagging eyelids, nothing ages you more quickly than sagging eyebrows. In fact, sagging eyebrows can even alter your expression.

A sagging brow occurs for the same reason that this type of problem occurs in other parts of our body—as we age, every bit of our bodies tends to sag a little bit. This is because of the way our fat thins or is redistributed, the effects of gravity, and also the deterioration of elastin, the substance found in our skin that, along with collagen, gives it elasticity.

Once we lose the elastin, things don't bounce back the way they used to. Our brow becomes heavy. The fat that collects in that area and the heaviness of it make our eyes look tired and heavy. This can cause puffiness and loose skin on the eyelid, and it can alter your expression because the shape of your eyebrow drastically changes.

In the old days, the brow was lifted surgically. This can still be done, and is often needed for those in their fifties, sixties, and older, or even for younger people who have a severely sagging brow. A brow lift is an invasive procedure and the recovery time can take several days to weeks. In many cases, doing a brow lift with simple BOTOX injections is the better way to go.

How does it work? Consider that your eyebrow is like a marionette, controlled by several strings. These strings are your muscles, which even when relaxed, are still under slight tension. They are, in fact, under about a 40 percent contraction. With BOTOX, however, the muscles are under no tension, so lines stretch out. By using BOTOX on these muscles selectively, your dermatologic surgeon can change the shape of the brow and add more of an arch. Most people are completely satisfied with this. However, those in their fifties, sixties, and older, or even those who are younger but have a severe sagging brow, may need a more traditional brow lift. This is performed either surgically, by making an incision along the hairline and removing the loose skin, or by removing skin above the eyebrow, which can leave a minimal scar.

# dark circles: lighten up

If you've got dark circles under your eyes, you look not only sleep deprived, but you may also look haggard and older. This is a frustrating problem because usually nothing is further from the truth. You can be completely rested yet dogged by these circles.

Even worse, you might be quite young. Dark circles can appear surprisingly early, thanks to heredity. We've not only seen people in their twenties with this problem but occasionally we've even seen them in their teens.

These deep circles stem from a combination of causes. First, as you get older, the skin under your eye thins, and this causes the vasculature—or veins and blood vessels beneath it—to show through. Also, pigment in the skin can change and become darker. In addition, as you wrinkle, this creates lines under your eyes, and with lines come shadows. All these combine to make the area underneath your eye appear darker.

Because dark rings develop from different causes, a combination of methods that use filling and laser resurfacing is usually needed to lighten them. In addition, if the darkness is caused by hereditary changes in pigmentation, bleaching agents can be used.

## filling

As we've discussed in other parts of this book, as we age, we lose the superficial fat layer under the skin, making our facial features more pronounced. This is also true of the area under the eye. One way to lighten this dark area is to fill it, ideally with your own fat, which has been harvested from another area. Filling substances such as collagen or Restylane may also be used.

But just filling in the area isn't enough. Because darker pigment or blood vessels show through, and there are also lines, laser resurfacing is also a good idea. Which resurfacing laser to choose? One treatment with a YAG or other laser to target the vessels doesn't usually work that well. However, resurfacing with a $CO_2$ laser under the eyes, even though the downtime is five to seven days, usually pays off with great tightening results. But as we noted in chapter 6, don't undergo a $CO_2$ laser resurfacing procedure piecemeal. Doing the area under the eyes, the crow's-feet, or the lines around the upper lid is fine because these areas, shadowed by your eye and your nose from sun exposure, generally look lighter than the rest of your face anyway. But doing only other specific areas can result in unwanted lighter patches on your face. That's why $CO_2$ laser resurfacing should be performed on the whole face, or only in these specific areas just mentioned.

After this refilling and laser resurfacing treatment is done, a bleaching agent may be applied just to make sure that the dark pigment does not return. Bleaching agents, which are applied as a cream, are also sometimes used to lighten dark spots on the skin.

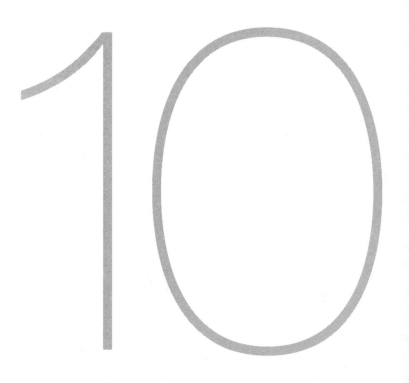

# 10

## HAIR TODAY *AND*

## TOMORROW

Barry didn't mind, many years ago, when his hair turned white. In fact, with his twinkling blue eyes, his white hair made him resemble Paul Newman a bit. But he was alarmed when as he neared sixty, his flowing locks began thinning. This came about when he was newly divorced and dating for the first time in decades. "Just when I'm getting out dating again I'm faced with the prospect of becoming bald. I'd better ask my doctor for a Viagra-Rogaine cocktail," he joked.

Actually, Barry was joking about the Viagra. But we can help him with his hair loss. Perhaps Rogaine is, or isn't, his best choice. When it comes to hair restoration, there are lots of options these days.

Ideal body shapes and weights change throughout the years, but the desire for hair on our heads does not. We remain a society obsessed with hair. Yet baldness is one of our most vexing problems.

For centuries, we have been trying to relieve ourselves of our genetic propensity to shed our hair. We've tried many ways—and failed numerous times.

Radiation, elixirs, salves, mechanical stimulation (massage, vibration)—the follicularly weak have tried all these methods yet failed in their sheer hope to sprout any growth. And that doesn't even take in all the other attempts, ranging from toupees to combovers, which have subjected many of their wearers to ridicule.

Still, baldness is prevalent among both men and women. But today there are proven methods that can restore hair. Best of all, there are a variety of hair restoration treatments that can fit anyone, no matter what their age.

For instance Matt, a thirty-eight-year-old investment banker, doesn't fit anyone's idea of an "old, balding man." He's in good shape and he works hard at it. But over the past five years, he's noticed his hair getting progressively thinner. He's also noticed his coworkers' eyes stray occasionally to his hairline when they're talking to him. To compensate, he cuts his hair short, but he prefers to wear it longer. Because he takes pride in his appearance he would like to maintain and restore some of the hair he had in his youth. Matt tried Rogaine (minoxidil) without success. But he's far from out of options. Matt is a great candidate for Propecia (finasteride). This oral medication will help him keep the hair he has left. Then hair restoration surgery can thicken the hair along his hairline. He can grow his hair longer, style it any way he chooses, and his hair will look perfectly natural. The bonus—he won't need to lose any time from work, and since the hair restoration will be a gradual process, his coworkers won't even notice that he's had anything done.

# hair loss

## the myths versus the truth

To take advantage of today's hair-loss remedies, you have to change your thinking. The first step is to learn the truth, not the myths, about hair loss. Here are the most popular myths:

- If there is baldness on your mother's side of the family, you are doomed: Actually, hair loss does not come from only the mother's side of the family. As with most genetic traits, there is often a predictable yet sometimes surprising course of genetic hand-me-downs that reflects the traits of both parents and their extended families. And the severity of that baldness can range drastically.

- Stress causes hair loss: Actually, it doesn't.

- Hair loss is due to a deficiency: No, it isn't, so vitamins, herbs, and other supplements are truly a waste of money.

- The way you treat your hair causes baldness: Blow-drying, styling, and using different types of shampoos, conditioners, hair gels, sprays, and other hair products have no effect on the cause, speed of growth, or on the ability to prevent hair loss.

## types of hair loss

All of us have 150,000 hairs on our head, busily growing, resting, and shedding. Yes, we shed our hair like animals do. But unlike other animals, which shed all their hair at one time, we do not. Approximately 85 percent of our hair grows while 12 percent rests, and 3 percent sheds.

We naturally shed about 150 hairs a day when we are not losing hair, so finding some stray hairs in the sink or in a hairbrush is perfectly normal.

However, there are abnormal types of hair loss. These are sudden hair loss, baldness (in men), and hair thinning (in women).

## sudden hair loss

If you are losing your hair, you are probably becoming bald (if you are a man) or your hair is thinning (if you are a woman). But if you suddenly find yourself losing a surprising amount of hair, this might not be the case; you might be suffering from sudden hair loss, which may be a medical problem.

Sudden hair loss, medically known as telogen effluvium, occurs in a previously normal scalp. The hair loss is diffuse and doesn't cause patches. You can lose a considerable portion of your hair before you even notice it.

Telogen effluvium can occur because of several reasons, including:

- Hormonal changes following giving birth
- Malnutrition due to severe dieting
- Severe illness
- Major surgery requiring general anesthesia
- Certain medications, including some cardiac medications and some antidepressants
- Chronic emotional stress

Many people can experience these changes without turning a hair, so to speak. But in others, the hair becomes "shocked" and suddenly stops growing, entering the resting phase. Then this resting hair all falls out at once. If this happens to you and you can't figure out the cause, talk to your doctor. Once the underlying cause is rooted out and resolved, your hair will begin growing normally.

## men: baldness

The medical term for what we commonly call "baldness" is androgenic alopecia (AGA). This is a genetic propensity that causes the hair follicles to shrink and shorten the growing cycle in response to circulating "male hormones" (hormones that are responsible for masculine characteristics) know as androgens (testosterone and dihydroxytestosterone [DHT], its active metabolite).

Over the years, usually starting in their twenties, some men's hair follicles, for a cause not clearly understood, develop a sensitivity to testosterone hormones (and possibly other factors as yet unknown) that causes this growing cycle to shorten. The hair becomes shorter and shorter and thinner and thinner until only peach fuzz exists and a permanent state of rest. The maximum length to which we can grow our hair is dependent on the length of the growth phase; Crystal Gayle has a very long growth phase; Yul Brynner had none. Why some people develop differences in this growing cycle is unknown. There doesn't seem to be any advantage of natural selection to be bald (excuse us, follicularly challenged).

Everyone, no matter how much or how little hair they seem

to have, develops some degree of AGA over time. If you examine the hair of people between eighteen and eighty, all will have a significant reduction of hair density. The decrease may not be noticeable, but it's there.

## women: "see-through hair"

Joyce is an attractive woman in her midfifties. She's always been known for her lovely auburn hair. Lately, though, Joyce has grown increasingly self-conscious. She's quick to take the elevator instead of the stairs because she knows that, if seen from a certain angle in the back, her hair is so thin that her scalp peeks through. Lately she's taken to wearing scarves; it's fine in the winter, she figures, although she's wondering what she'll do when summer comes. "What's next?" she asks herself wryly. "A kiddie's sailor cap?"

The major myth about baldness is the belief that only men get bald. AGA affects just as many women as it does men. This is because women have not only female sex hormones but androgens as well. This is a reason why women get acne, which is another androgen-based condition.

But there is a difference between women and men when it comes to hair loss. Men can get a receding hairline and an actual bald spot. Men also develop hair loss earlier, beginning in their twenties and thirties, while women usually develop it after menopause (although sometimes it can occur earlier).

Women, on the other hand (although there are exceptions), maintain their hairlines but develop diffuse thinning or "see-through hair." If a woman starts out with very thick hair, it may thin out unnoticeably to other people. But women who start out with thin hair can develop "see-through hair."

Why do these gender differences exist? Again, we don't know. But for women too, the hair in the back of the head is generally protected from thinning. This is why hair transplantation, discussed later, works so well.

# medications

Over the past twenty years, great strides have been made in both hair-loss prevention and hair restoration.

First came Rogaine (minoxidil). This was the first FDA-approved medication for hair loss. While taking the drug (developed to treat severe hypertension), some patients noticed that hair began growing on their scalps. So a topical version was developed to treat hair loss. It's been found to have some effect on hair loss, mostly in the back of the scalp. Exactly how Rogaine works isn't known, but the effect is believed to be related to the increased blood supply provided to the follicles. Over the years, a 5 percent extrastrength treatment was developed for men, and a 2 percent solution for women was marketed. When a generic form of the drug became available, the cost dropped sharply. The regular-strength formula now costs about $10 a month.

But just because Rogaine is FDA approved doesn't mean it has a dramatic effect. Rogaine must be used twice daily, it's a bit oily, and to maintain its effect it must be used forever—or until you tire of it. Rogaine also must be used for about four months before you notice any effects at all. If you stop using it, your hair—or lack thereof—will revert back to its original state.

The consensus is that Rogaine works great for very few people and does do a little to maintain or restore hair in many, but it does make a good supplement to some other treatments now available. But for a significant number of people it only makes their thin hair oily. Rogaine's side effects range from none to mild to moderate irritation and itching. In rare cases, users experience hair growth in areas where it's unwanted, such as the face.

The breakthrough in hair-loss medication came with the advent of Propecia (finasteride). Marketed under the name Proscar, finasteride was used for prostate enlargement, and as with Rogaine, hair growth was noted as a side effect. This is not surprising, because finasteride blocks conversion of one form of testosterone to the more active form (DHT). Since the more active form is decreased, so is hair loss.

Propecia is dramatically effective. Our experience with our patients confirms studies showing that about 80 to 90 percent of those taking Propecia maintain stable hair counts over the years, and about 50 to 60 percent experience some degree of regrowth. This is a breakthrough.

But although the drug has been used for almost two decades, we are uncertain whether these positive effects on hair loss will last indefinitely. Though the drug inhibits a hormone, this is not really a cause for concern. Only the production of DHT is blocked, leaving most of the body's other hormonal functions untouched.

When Propecia first came on the market, a lot was written

about its sexual side effects (decreased libido, erectile dysfunction, or decreased sperm count). This potential problem was overblown; studies find that only about 2 percent of individuals experience sexual side effects. However, research also finds that about 1.3 percent of the participants who took a placebo (sugar pill) also suffered similar side effects. So the problem is almost negligible. In our practice, we've found this drug is well tolerated with minimal side effects over time, and if they do occur, they disappear over time or once the drug is stopped.

Propecia is taken in pill form once daily. The earlier you start taking it, the better. A thirty-year-old man with generally thinning but significant hair counts is the best candidate for maintaining his hair and even regrowing some of it. A fellow who is a fifty-year-old cue ball is going to need more than a pill to stimulate those hair follicles. However, once you stop taking Propecia, your hair (or lack thereof) will go back to being how it originally was if you had never taken the drug.

Unfortunately, women of childbearing age cannot take Propecia because it can cause birth defects. Postmenopausal females and younger women who cannot bear children have taken the drug with mixed results. However, there is a medication that may be of help to these women. This is spironolactone, which helps reduce the hormone testosterone, which is present in women, although in smaller amounts than in men.

Although it is not the same as taking an oral pill, such as Propecia, or applying a topical preparation, like Rogaine, some men may benefit from scalp injections containing a low-dose steroid. This has helped halt hair loss in some men.

# modern hair restoration: not your father's hair transplant

When hair transplant surgery was introduced in the 1950s you could easily spot it. The results weren't that much of an improvement over a toupee, which looked pretty much like a Davy Crockett hat perched atop the unhappy head. To create this unfortunate look, bunches of hairs were taken from the back of the head and transplanted into round holes in the bald area. These unnatural-looking large "plugs" gave the unfortunate wearer a "cornrow appearance" that was easily recognizable as being a hair transplant. The bald areas were covered with hair, but the hairlines still looked phony, so the men had to comb their hair over or forward. Plugs weren't considered to be any better than the unfortunate toupee. But with today's advances, the only noticeable hair transplants are bad hair transplants.

By mimicking the natural idiosyncrasies and asymmetries of hairlines and the patterns of hair growth in different areas of the scalp, we can now create natural-appearing hair that grows and can be styled or blow-dried. These are full heads of hair that require no maintenance, do not lose their effect over time, and entail minimal discomfort to acquire.

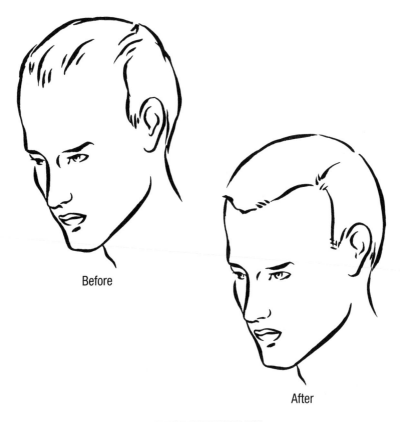

Before

After

HAIR TRANSPLANTATION FOR MEN

## not for men only

Hair restoration surgery is often thought of as "for men only," but the procedure is easily done in women, sometimes even more effectively. This is because of the female pattern of hair loss. The totally bald spots men have can be difficult to fill in without its being noticeable, but since a woman's hair generally only thins, the cosmetic effect of hair replacement can be dramatically attractive.

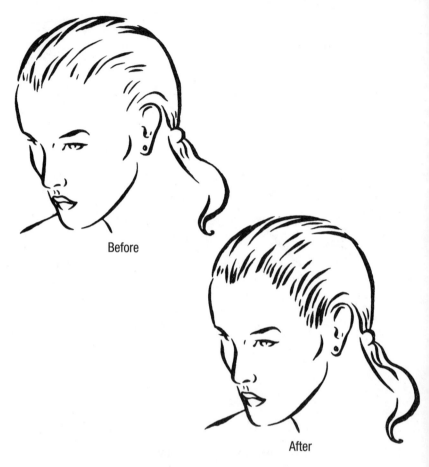

Before

After

HAIR TRANSPLANTATION FOR WOMEN

## why transplants work

Hair is genetically programmed at the root or hair follicle, and some hair lasts for a lifetime. The success of hair transplantation depends on the fact that transplanted hair follicles (roots moved from their original location to another area) will behave as they would have in their original donor site. This is the big advantage of hair transplantation: it's your own hair! It will grow, cut, and style exactly like the hair on the back of your head does—the hair from which the grafts came. So if a hair transplantation procedure is done well, we defy anyone to tell the difference between the grafted hair and the hair growing on the back of your head.

## how transplants work

For a hair transplant, small donor strips of hair-bearing scalp are removed from the back and sides of the head. They are divided into grafts for placement into the balding areas. These hair-bearing grafts are carefully inserted into small holes or slits that are made in the balding scalp, often with a laser. The grafts can also be inserted among existing hairs to increase their density and thicken the area.

## frequently asked questions about hair transplantation

q: Who should do the hair transplant?

a: As with many of the techniques described in this book, the success of a hair transplant is highly dependent on the practitioner, so you should choose your physician with care. Hair transplantation was developed and refined by dermatologists, so many specialize in this area.

Be certain to find a qualified dermatological surgeon to do the transplant. Some of the criteria are the same as those you would use when seeking a doctor to do other types of cosmetic procedures, including finding a physician who is board certified, has considerable experience in hair transplantation, and charges reasonable but not bargain-basement fees. Also make sure the physician is experienced with all the different types of hair grafting discussed in this chapter.

Because hair transplantation is a labor-intensive procedure, the physician performing it works with a team of medical assistants. You should make certain ahead of time that the physician will be present at all times during the transplant procedure. You should also meet and feel comfortable with some of the other team members as well. The physician performs all of the surgical steps, including the designing of the hairline. The assistants help the physician remove and harvest the hair from the back of the head, prepare the hair for transplantation, and insert it into the new hairline.

q: What is hair transplantation like?

a: Hair transplantation is an in-office procedure that is done under local anesthetic. You can go back to work the next day, although you should wear a hat or other type of head covering for about a week.

During the procedure, which takes four to five hours, you'll be awake and comfortable, so you can talk, read the paper, or even watch a movie. The only thing you'll feel during the procedure is pinpricks in your scalp at the beginning because that is where the anesthesia is injected. The anesthesia lasts into the evening, so this is, in effect, a pain-free procedure, and patients rarely need anything stronger than Tylenol. You'll wear a turban for the first twenty-four hours. After forty-eight to seventy-two hours, you can gently wash your hair, taking caution to avoid the healing hairs. Uncommon complications include temporary swelling or black eyes, which can develop from any surgery on the scalp. Scabs at the sites of the hair placement develop and fall out in seven to ten days. During that time, the hair can be styled to cover the healing area. Stitches in the back of the scalp are removed in a week. It's a good idea to keep your hair a little long in the back to camouflage the stitches until they are removed.

Bear in mind that this is a process that takes patience on your part. After the stitches are removed, you will see basically . . . nothing. You'll have a very thin, barely noticeable scar in the back of your head with no sign of growth and no noticeable signs of anything having been done to you on the front of your head. Nothing—zero—will happen for about three or four months. Then, just when you're thinking that you're the only person that the procedure won't work for, tiny hairs will suddenly begin growing out of the grafted sites. Over the next few months, the hair will begin developing some length and the increased thickness will become truly noticeable. But we believe the final results cannot be truly seen until six months to a year after the procedure.

Hair transplantation can cost anywhere from $4,000 to $8,000 a session. Some doctors charge per graft.

# minigrafts and micrografts

Over the years, the size of the grafts has become smaller and finer. Now minigrafts and micrografts are being used, providing even easier procedures and more natural results. Minigrafts contain three to seven hairs and micrografts have one to three hairs.

Thanks to improved techniques, the surgeon can make most efficient use of the donor area while providing the best cosmetic result in this area. The introduction of smaller grafts has afforded tremendous flexibility in distributing natural hair evenly. The new grafts contain between one and five hairs. At the front of the hairline, for instance, the surgeon can use a single hair and two hair grafts in the front and then grafts with greater hairs as you go back. This produces a soft, natural hairline. Minigrafts and micrografts are also less noticeable and heal faster during the initial period following transplantation. Large numbers of grafts can be done in each session to give you a natural look as quickly as possible.

For women, micrografting is an especially well-suited technique because hair can be grafted in between thinning areas without removing any potentially viable hairs. This increases hair density without sacrificing any hair at all. The sizes and shapes of the grafts can be varied as required to increase the overall fullness.

# scalp reduction

Hair transplantation alone, however, cannot always provide the desired coverage, particularly for those patients who are experiencing more extensive forms of baldness. In such cases, hair transplantation can be combined with other techniques to provide the coverage and density necessary. Scalp reduction involves reducing the area of the bald scalp by surgical excision, then pulling upward and lifting the hair-bearing skin together. This decreases the size of the bald patch.

Scalp reductions are helpful for patients whose bald area is too large for the donor hair on the back of the head to supply enough grafts. For a scalp reduction, the bald spot is cut out and the skin sewn back together without the need for hair from the back of the head. This allows more efficient use of an irreplaceable commodity: the donor hair.

## laser surgery

The $CO_2$ laser is sometimes used to produce the recipient sites for the grafts. Studies to determine if there is better hair growth and healing using this instrument show mixed results. We generally do not prefer this technique.

*turn-back-the-clock tip*

Okay, we know we are becoming a broken record (or scratched CD) about this, but we can't help but reiterate that the best results for hair restoration, as with other cosmetic-enhancing techniques, are often achieved through a combination of methods. For instance, Rogaine or Propecia are often used in conjunction with surgical hair transplantation to produce excellent results.

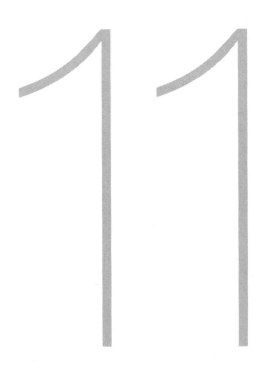

# 11

## ROAD MAPS ARE

## GREAT — BUT NOT ON

## YOUR LEGS

Kelly flipped through the racks in the dress store and spotted the perfect outfit. With its short, flirty skirt it was exactly what she had been looking for. Then she remembered, and her heart sank. A few years ago, it would have been perfect. But Kelly was forty-four, and her legs, once her best asset, were marred with bulging, purplish veins. With tears in her eyes, she hung the dress back on the rack.

## varicose veins

Varicose veins are twisted, distended veins located just beneath the skin and are most often obvious on the legs. Although we tend to focus only on how ugly they look, these veins are also the most common cause of undiagnosed leg pain in women.

The cause of varicose veins is the unfortunate effect of gravity. We have two systems of veins that carry blood to the heart. These are the deep veins, which lie deep in the muscles and carry most of the blood, and the superficial, or surface, veins, which are often visible just under the skin and in the fat.

When our blood circulates throughout the body, these vein systems collect it and pump it upward, against the force of gravity, to the heart. These two vein systems are connected by valves that keep the blood flowing smoothly. These valves can, over time, break down. When this occurs, the visible results are varicose veins.

Varicose veins are common, especially in women. Several risk factors may make some people more susceptible to them, including:

- Family history. If one or both of your parents had this problem, you're more likely to.

- Gender. Women get varicose veins two to four times as often as men do. Hormonal fluctuations before and after pregnancy and at menopause are the causes. But the treatments described here can help either gender.

- Estrogen and/or birth control pills.

- Prolonged standing or sitting.

- Tight girdles or garter belts.

- Injury to the leg.

## prevention

As long as we're earthbound, we'll always have gravity to contend with, so this problem will always be with us. But if you want to prevent varicose veins, follow these smart steps:

- Choose nonimpact exercises like cycling, walking, rowing, and swimming. They may be useful because they pump blood out of your legs and back toward your heart.

- Swim if at all possible. It may be especially beneficial, since the mild water pressure on your legs drives blood out of the superficial veins. In addition, swimming puts your legs at the same level as your heart, further reducing pressure on your leg veins and valves.

- Don't gain excess weight or fluctuate in weight—this stresses the veins (and the rest of your body, for that matter).

- Elevate your legs whenever possible and when you sleep.

- Wear low-heeled shoes.

- Wear medically prescribed support hose or tight commercial support hose.

*turn-back-the-clock tip*

As with everything else in this book, the best time to start paying attention to these problems is sooner rather than later. Waiting until hundreds of these vessels develop makes it extremely difficult to deal with the problem. Starting to prevent and treat them when you are young is the best strategy.

## treatments

Fortunately, we don't need these superficial vessels for survival, so we can treat the problem by just removing them.

In the past, the major way of removing varicose veins was by vein stripping, an invasive surgery that required hospitalization, general anesthesia, and a considerable recovery period. But over the past ten years other techniques have been developed that make this seem archaic.

These forms of treatment are sclerotherapy, ambulatory phlebectomy, and laser or pulsed light therapy.

## sclerotherapy

Sclerotherapy is a safe and virtually painless nonsurgical procedure. The process is accomplished by injecting the vessels with a mild sclerosing (irritating) solution. This solution causes irritation in the vein wall and stimulates the natural cleansing action of your body to eventually absorb the vessel. Within three weeks to six months, the offending vessel virtually disappears. Blood flow is also shifted to healthy veins nearby. This procedure improves not only the appearance your legs but also the circulation of blood within them as well.

Sclerotherapy is most successful on red, purple, and bluish superficial veins and requires patience on your part. Several treatments spaced four to six weeks apart are usually necessary. The vessel can take from a few weeks to six months to disappear, and varicose veins can return with time or lack of prevention. On the other hand, there's no downtime after treatment; you can resume your normal activities immediately.

If you decide on sclerotherapy, you should know what type of agent your doctor will use. There are two popular agents. One is hypertonic saline, which is basically concentrated salt water. It is readily available and relatively cheap. Unfortunately, though, it causes significant cramping when it's injected and can cause pigment changes along the treated vessel, and there's a chance of developing ulcers (an open sore on the leg) if the fluid is accidentally placed outside the vessel in the skin. Sotradecol, another popular agent, is far less painful and more effective, but it can also cause leg ulcers and is expensive. The cost of sclerotherapy ranges dramatically depending on the agent used and on the number and size of the veins treated at one time. One treatment can be anywhere from $100 to $400 a session.

## ambulatory phlebectomy

Ambulatory phlebectomy is a minimally invasive procedure that has largely replaced the much more drastic hospital-based surgery known as vein stripping. Only in the most extreme circumstances of varicosities is the traditional stripping or similar techniques used.

Ambulatory phlebectomy is especially good for removing the larger blue and deep colorless vessels. This procedure is done in the doctor's office. Since local anesthesia is used, you are awake but pain free and comfortable during the entire procedure.

First, the doctor uses a simple handheld ultrasound device to trace out the vein to be removed. Then the doctor makes a series of barely detectable pinpoint incisions along the track of the vessel and teases them out. After all the veins are removed, a process that takes thirty to sixty minutes, your leg is tightly wrapped with an Ace bandage and you're told to get up and walk around the office for twenty minutes before going home. You'll wear a sup-

Before
After

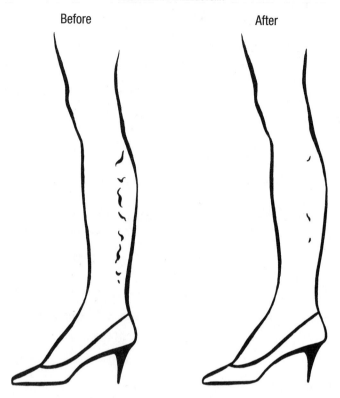

port stocking for two weeks after surgery, and you can resume
your normal activities immediately.

A number of variations on this procedure have been devised,
using radio frequencies and a laser to destroy the vessel from the
inside, but ambulatory phlebectomy continues to offer the sim-
plest, most straightforward answer for removing large varicose
veins. Side effects include mild bruising, small scars, and a small
chance of superficial infections.

Ambulatory phlebectomy gets to the root of the problem by

removing the larger vessels with the broken valves that eventually cause the smaller red and purple vessels. With this process, you can nip in the bud (or in the vessel, so to speak) the development of a whole array of cosmetically displeasing blood vessels.

## lasers and similar devices

Because we live in a gadget-focused society, we too often assume that *Star Wars* technology is the best choice for effective medical treatments. Sure, use of lasers and other pulsed light devices sounds appealing. But although there have been great strides in this technology, we believe that the use of lasers and light sources in the treatment of leg veins is premature.

There is a role for laser and light-source therapy, however. Many people with varicose veins also have spider veins. Spider veins mar the appearance of the legs. These vessels, known medically as telangiectasia, are dot-size red patches of skin with small blood vessels radiating outward, like a spider. Often these vessels are too small for doctors to inject with sclerosants. Spider veins can be removed with a series of laser treatments anywhere on the body. The potential risks are similar to sclerotherapy, including bruising and infection.

As with many cosmetic procedures, there is sometimes no ideal treatment. In most cases in which a wide variety of vessel types exist in one patient, stubborn, large varicose veins can be treated using sclerotherapy and ambulatory phlebectomy while laser treatments can be used to "clean up" the most superficial of vessels. Once again, a combined approach of minimally invasive treatments usually offers the best results.

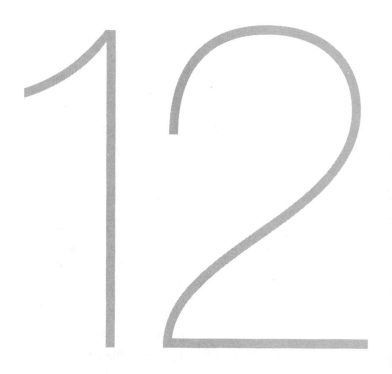

# 12

## OUT DAMNED SPOT:

## BENIGN GROWTH

## REMOVAL

Samantha's appearance was marred when an unsightly mole popped up on the end of her nose. Images of a warty, hook-nosed Halloween witch sprang into her mind. She tried in vain to cover it with makeup but couldn't mask its shape. She assumed she'd have to live with it, when a chance discussion with a dermatologist she met in passing changed her mind. "What's that on your nose?" the dermatologist asked. Samantha was mortified. But her embarrassment turned to relief when the physician said, "What are you doing with that mole on your nose? That can be very easily removed." And, poof—after one office visit, Samantha the Witch was transformed back into Samantha the Princess.

Well, it was sort of like that. The point is, you don't have to suffer with unsightly moles, cysts, or growths. But many people suffer self-consciously with these problems because they don't realize how easily they can be remedied.

Many blemishes that occur on the skin, such as age or liver spots, birthmarks, moles, warts, cysts, and scars, can be eliminated or at least improved by an appropriate dermatological surgical procedure. The removal of birthmarks, wrinkles, and age spots is covered in other chapters of this book. But that still leaves moles, benign growths, skin lesions, and cysts. Generally, these can be removed without pain or risk in an office visit.

As you'll see, there are different methods that can be used to remove benign growths, or lesions. How to remove them depends on the type of lesion as well as their size and location on the body.

The methods include:

- Shaving (this can also be done to remove moles).

- Surgical excision—cutting into the skin, removing the growth, and then stitching up the wound.

- Desiccation and Curettage—the desiccation is done with an electric machine that cauterizes, or lightly burns, the area. *Curettage* refers to the scraping away of the benign growth.

- Subcision—a surgical way of improving the appearance of scars by detaching top skin tissue from scar tissue that is pulling it down.

- Chemical ablation—refers to burning off the area with a chemical acid or base. In this case, liquid nitrogen is sprayed onto the tissue, which freezes it, and the growth falls off.

In addition, cysts can be popped out, as you'll see, and liposuction can be used to remove benign fatty tumors. Physicians have a host of techniques at their disposal.

# moles

A mole is a small, usually dark skin growth that develops from the pigment-producing cells in the skin. Depending on their location and appearance, moles can be considered either desirable (beauty marks) or unsightly.

Since it's common knowledge that melanoma, the lethal form of skin cancer, arises from moles, many people erroneously assume that all moles are "bad" and therefore must be removed. This isn't true; it's normal for people to have twenty to forty moles on their body. Still, you should bring suspicious-looking moles to the attention of a dermatologist. Sometimes moles should be removed to prevent them from enlarging or becoming cancerous. A change in a mole can indicate a serious problem (see chapter 14).

Benign moles are the most common skin growths that people have removed. These are small, circular growths that can be brown or clear. They can appear on the skin and also on the scalp.

Even though a benign mole poses no danger, it can be unattractive or can become irritated by clothing or make shaving difficult. Sometimes, moles crop up unattractively on the tip of the nose. Hair may even spring out of large moles on the cheek. In this case, a person might very well choose to have the mole removed.

Moles can generally be taken care of in an office visit. The physician will shave off the raised mole flush with the surrounding skin. This process will form a scab, then turn pink, and then heal. The healing process takes about a week.

Shaving is the treatment of choice for permanently removing the vast majority of moles—about 98 percent. In the rare event that the mole reappears, it can then be excised or cut away. This will require a few stitches and will leave a thin, permanent scar line. If hair grows out of a mole, the mole itself may not need to be removed; the hair can be eliminated with electrolysis.

## cysts

Cysts are small closed sacs filled with secretions that come from the skin but have become blocked. Cysts can be genetic or can occur on the scalp when hair follicles become blocked; some unfortunate individuals have hundreds on the scalp. If a cyst is infected, the dermatologist must drain the contents before removing the sac. Often, though, the dermatologist makes a small hole and pops the whole cyst out. Sometimes even large cysts can be removed in this fashion, almost like the way a baby is delivered through a relatively small opening. Depending on the size of the opening made, the site may or may not be closed with stitches.

## earlobe repair and reduction

Although it doesn't come under the heading of "growth removal," another surgical procedure that dermatologists are called upon to perform is earlobe repair. Obviously, wearing pierced earrings is very common—for both men and women. Sometimes wearing heavy earrings or catching a hoop tears through the earlobe. Or the hole becomes elongated and unattractive. Sometimes, with age, the ear remains a normal size but the lobe grows. In all these cases, earlobes can be easily repaired, reduced in size, or even plumped up. Ripped-through holes in earlobes can be surgically repaired. When an earlobe is repaired, it can be surgically decreased in size. Filling material can be used to fill the earlobe and make it plumper and younger looking. The $CO_2$ laser can also be used to make an earlobe thicker. This is because, as we grow older, the amount of collagen in our earlobes decreases. Laser treatment thickens the collagen and tightens the skin, making the earlobe fuller. Using a filling treatment, such as fat, can also replace lost connective tissue and make the earlobe fuller.

## keratoses

There are two kinds of keratoses: actinic and seborrheic.

Actinic keratoses are thick, warty, rough, reddish growths that appear on the sun-exposed areas of the body. These growths can be removed through chemical peeling and are discussed in chapter 5.

Seborrheic keratoses are raised, flesh-colored, tan, or brown growths that can appear anywhere on the skin. They often become itchy and irritated by clothing. They are most common in middle-aged and older people. They resemble barnacles, and we've heard them referred to as the "barnacles of aging." These growths aren't cancerous and don't become so, but they can be aesthetically undesirable. They can be easily removed surgically.

## lipomas

Lipomas are soft deposits of fatty material that grow under the skin, causing round or oval lumps. Lipomas are more common in women than in men, and although they can develop anywhere on the body, they are most commonly found on the forearms, torso, and back of the neck. These are benign tumors, or growths, of fatty tissue. Lipomas usually don't require treatment, but they can be unsightly. They can be removed using a small or large incision, depending on their size.

## acne scars

If the scar is deep, the punch graft method is used. This means that a cylindrical instrument is used to punch out the scar. The area is filled in with a graft taken with a slightly larger punch from behind the ear. Then dermabrasion, laser or collagen is used to smooth it. This is done under local anesthesia. The graft "takes" within 24 hours and subsequently heals as a much smoother scar.

## other scars

As we go through life, many things can create scars on our skin, ranging from accidents to surgery. Some scars are small but unattractive; others, like scars from heart bypass surgery, are large. There are cosmetic procedures to make these scars less noticeable.

For instance, many scars look bad because they appear always to be red, even when they are no longer fresh. Treatment with the Pulsed-dye laser, which removes red blood vessels, can make these scars far less angry looking.

Sometimes scars can be particularly ugly, especially if they grow thick. Thick scars that stay within the boundary of the injury or incision are called hypertrophic scars. Scarring that extends outside the boundary are called keloids. Such thickened scars lying above the skin can be smoothed out with cortisone injections and also treated with a laser.

This is what happened in Anne's case. Anne broke her arm in an accident and was sewn up in the emergency room. Because of her other injuries, the doctors couldn't spend much time making sure Anne's scar would be cosmetically perfect, and sure enough, it was far from it. So Anne turned to cosmetic surgery for help. Her scar was smoothed out by a cortisone injection, and the ugly redness was taken care of with the Pulsed-dye laser. Also, the jagged part of the scar was cut and resewn skillfully. Her arm now sports a barely noticeable, evenly colored thin line as opposed to a jagged, thick scar.

## warts

Warts are caused by a virus and consist of piled-up layers of skin. Warts may develop on people of all ages anywhere on the skin. Some warts require cryosurgery, electrosurgery and curettage, or laser surgery. Cryosurgery is done using a spray of liquid nitrogen. It's best used for large warts on the fingers, palms, or soles. This is not a good choice for those with even slightly dark skin because this substance may remove pigment. If the wart recurs, and you don't want to undergo another liquid nitrogen treatment, or if you have darker skin, electrosurgery with curettage is a better option. Electrosurgery is performed to destroy the scar, and curettage means scraping it off. Pulsed-dye lasers can also be used to destroy warts, but it is more expensive and may not be any better than electrosurgery and curettage.

part 2

# What You Can Do for Yourself

# 13

## ENHANCE YOUR

## BEAUTY RIGHT NOW

Our mission is to help you turn back the clock. The treatments we've discussed can accomplish this. But there are things you can do to enhance your appearance. Also, once you have cosmetic procedures done, the steps covered in this chapter will help you protect your investment.

Preventative skin care can help you look younger longer. If you follow these steps yourself, they will help, although they may not accomplish all you desire. If you do them in conjunction with undergoing cosmetic procedures, you'll get the best possible results. After all, the last thing you want is to carelessly undo what you've so painstakingly had done. If you pay for a laser peel and many of your wrinkles disappear, what good does that do if you continue to smoke and bake in the sun. New ones will appear!

# enhance your appearance without cosmetic surgery

There are many ways you can enhance your entire appearance without a bit of cosmetic surgery. Here are some ideas.

- Make sure your hair is the best color and style for you. There's never been a better time to experiment with hair color, either permanent or temporary. A visit to a skilled hairstylist can help you choose the best look for your hair. As you grow older, keep your hair and eyebrows a shade lighter. This makes the lines on your face less noticeable.

- Make sure your wardrobe is flattering and that your shoes and other accessories are up-to-date. Weed your closet annually to get rid of outmoded clothing.

- Make sure your teeth are in good shape. Considering the abuse we put our teeth through, it's a wonder they hold up as well as they do. Organic pigments build up over time, causing discoloration. Coffee, tea, and smoking stain the teeth. Certain medications, such as the antibiotic tetracycline, which is prescribed for infections, can cause stains as well. Cosmetic dentistry offers many procedures now to whiten teeth, but you can also try one of the at-home bleaching kits on the market.

- Squinting can cause wrinkles to form around your eyes. Always be sure that you're wearing the right prescription contacts, glasses, and/or sunglasses.

- Don't forget to smile. That pensive, moody look might look alluring on a young person, but dour on you. Want proof? If you're among the many who hate their driver's license picture, smile the next time you have it taken. You'll be surprised at the difference.

## stop smoking

If you're a smoker, you're probably tired of hearing about the harm you're doing to your health. Smoking is to blame for a host of diseases, including lung cancer (which kills twenty thousand more women annually than does breast cancer), heart disease, stroke, osteoporosis, and more. But if that hasn't convinced you to quit, try looking in the mirror. Research studies show a strong connection between smoking and getting wrinkles. When you smoke your blood circulates less effectively, causing less blood to reach your skin. This results in the accelerated degeneration of the skin proteins collagen and elastin, ultimately resulting in wrinkles.

It's easy to say "don't smoke"—the tough part is to do it. Researchers are finding that cigarette smoking may be even more likely to cause lung cancer in women than in men. Smoking may also be more addictive to women. So if you smoke, consider one of the nonsmoking nicotine replacement products or medications on the market. It's the best thing you can do for your health—and your skin.

## use sun protection

It isn't the years that wreak havoc on your skin; it's the sunlight you've been exposed to since birth. Ninety percent of the changes on your face, like wrinkles and brown spots, are now known to come not from aging but from accumulated sun damage. Need proof? Look at the underside of your arm or your buttocks. See how soft and wrinkle free the skin is? This is the look of skin that hasn't been exposed to the sun.

By this point in our lives, we've all suffered some sun damage. To learn how to protect your skin and minimize further damage, see chapter 14.

## eat healthfully

Does the food you eat affect your skin? For years, doctors and researchers have struggled with this question and there's still no definitive answer. The belief that eating too much chocolate or too much greasy food makes acne worse were once accepted as gospel, but research shows them to be old wives' tales. It's now believed that diet does not affect chronic skin conditions. In fact, most of these conditions, like acne, have more to do with imbalances in the patient's immune system and are governed much more by genetics than by what the patient eats or drinks.

Studies show that eating a healthy diet is essential for good health. But when it comes to your skin, there is no quick fix, like eating lots of carrots or downing handfuls of vitamins.

This isn't to say that some vitamins won't prove helpful. There is much interest in antioxidants, for instance, for the health of your skin and for your overall health as well. Antioxidant vitamins include vitamin C and E. It's believed these chemical compounds may help neutralize damage to your body's cells from substances it comes into contact with that are carcinogenic, or cancer promoting. Among these would be ultraviolet radiation from the sun. Indeed, studies have found these vitamins do have a subtle sun-protective effect, but they are not a substitute for the protective effects of sunscreen.

Also, there is some evidence that vitamins can affect your skin. Consider Accutane, for instance. Accutane is a very common drug used for acne. This is a potent drug and must be monitored closely. Accutane is derived from a source of vitamin A. In fact, since it is so potent, we tell patients taking it to avoid vitamin A. Other skin-effective substances derived from a source of vitamin A is the wrinkle-fighting topical cream Retin-A and retinol, its generic cousin.

So what's the bottom line? Despite some media reports and books to the contrary, there is no scientific evidence that the way you eat and the supplements you take can make you look younger, erase your wrinkles, or make your skin glow. But there is definite evidence that wise eating is a good way to maintain your ideal weight.

Keeping your weight in check is also important if you've had liposuction. Liposuction is a way to contour your body, not a way to lose weight. Liposuction also permanently removes fat cells from troublesome areas so they doesn't return. That is, under normal circumstances. If you do gain a great deal of weight after liposuction—say twenty pounds—you'll get fatter all over, including where you had the liposuction.

But too many of us—women especially—have become too terrified of food to even know how to eat a varied, healthful diet. You can bone up by following the U.S. Department of Agriculture's Dietary Guidelines for Americans, known as the Food Guide Pyramid. This eating plan stresses a healthy way of eating that is high in fiber and rich in fruits and vegetables. According to the Food Guide Pyramid, you should eat six to eleven daily servings of bread, cereal, rice, and pasta; three to five servings of vegetables; two to four servings of fruit; two to three servings of dairy foods; and two to three servings of protein foods, including meat, poultry, fish, dry beans, eggs, and nuts. Fats, oils, and sweets should be used sparingly.

You should also pay special attention to your diet to avoid osteoporosis, especially if you're a woman. Women, with their naturally thinner bones, are more likely to develop osteoporosis. Calcium helps keep bones strong. Dairy products are loaded with calcium. If you're watching your fat intake, low-fat dairy products have the same amount of calcium as the regular ones, and possibly more. Salmon, sardines, some breads and grain products, and certain vegetables, particularly broccoli, collard greens, and kale, are also rich in calcium. But it's virtually impossible to get enough calcium from food, so taking calcium supplements is recommended.

## don't forget exercise

Exercise is also important for looking and feeling younger than your years. After all, who wants a youthful face perched on a flabby body?

The results of a good exercise program are not instant, but they are worthwhile and long lasting. If you exercise and are happy with your body, this will enhance the effect of any procedures you chose to have done.

This is especially true if you've undergone liposuction. When you undergo liposuction, you are siphoning the fat out from under your skin, which is kind of like emptying air from a balloon. When that happens, a certain amount of laxity occurs, leaving the outer skin collapsed and wrinkled, pretty much like the outer layer of the deflated balloon. How much elasticity your body retains determines how good your liposuction result will be. If your body is toned, the results will look even better. So if you haven't toned up your body before the procedure, there is still time to begin afterward. When you tighten and build muscle underneath the skin, your body will look better and smoother when the skin retracts after liposuction. It takes about six months after the liposuction procedure to see the final result.

If you're undertaking a new exercise program, you should check with your physician first. Also, decide on the type of exercise that will benefit you the most.

There are three kinds of exercise:

- Aerobic—this type of exercise increases your endurance and the functioning of your heart and lungs. Examples include brisk walking, jogging, racewalking, swimming, bicycling (either stationary or on a real bicycle), and aerobic dancing.

- Strength building—this type of exercise builds up your muscles through the use of free weights or weight-training machines.

- Weight bearing—this type of exercise impacts the joints and is very valuable, especially for women, because it increases bone density and prevents osteoporosis. You can do both aerobic and weight-bearing exercises at the same time by choosing aerobic activities that apply some force to the bones, such as walking, jogging, aerobic dancing, and racquet sports.

By varying your workout to include these three types of exercise you'll reap the most benefits for the least amount of effort. The most important criterion of an exercise program is that you find it personally worthwhile. We all vary in our approaches. Some of us like to work out strenuously; others prefer to do activities they deem fun. Some of us like to exercise with a buddy, others prefer to do so alone. Whatever your choice, just remember that the most important thing about an exercise program is that you do it.

# bonus beauty tips

Here are some bonus beauty tips to help you look your best:

- Take a multivitamin daily. If you're female, add a calcium supplement, especially if you're past menopause. An iron supplement is beneficial prior to menopause.

- Rinsing your skin in salt water is good for it. The salt is antibacterial, exfoliates dead cells from your skin, and helps dry lesions.

- When you're choosing makeup, a green concealer gets rid of reddishness on your skin, while lilac helps mask black-and-bluish marks.

- Have your makeup done by a professional annually. This way you'll stay in touch with the latest makeup looks.

- As you grow older, your lips become thinner. Line your lips with lip liner slightly outside the shape of your actual lips; this prevents your lipstick from "bleeding."

- Apply a clear coat of nail polish on your nails each night to keep your nails looking good and prevent them from chipping.

- Use a "luminous" foundation or similar makeup product that reflects light; this makes blemishes less visible.

# troubleshooting guide: quick fixes for common problems

## acne

Acne, the most common skin condition, is due to the increase of hormones at adolescence. But although it occurs in all teenagers to some degree, it can also plague adults. It's not that unusual for people in their twenties, thirties, and very occasionally their forties to suffer from acne.

Here are some ways to treat and prevent mild acne. Serious acne requires the care of a dermatologist. Dermatologists can prescribe treatments, including the medication that cures acne, Accutane.

- The sun is good for acne, so enjoy it, but only in moderation. Use a gel or nongreasy sunscreen or sunblock.

- Use a mild nonsoap cleanser.

- Don't use a washcloth to scrub your face; it's too rough. Acne is not a problem of lack of cleanliness—it is deeper than that. Acne is caused by clogged hair follicles in your skin. In other words, think of a clogged drain; you can't unplug one by scrubbing the sink.

- Don't dry out your skin so much that you need a moisturizer.

- Use over-the-counter benzoyl peroxide products of 2½ to 5 percent strength. Start using this every three days and slowly increase to every night if possible. Don't let your skin get too dry, and stop if you develop a rash.

- To troubleshoot acne cysts that suddenly emerge, see Pimples or Acne Cysts, later in this chapter.

## aging skin

Aging skin is a term that encompasses wrinkles, lines, and a variety of lesions and marks that occur on our skin as we age. Much of this book contains information on how to help our skin age as gracefully as we do. These steps help prevent aging skin:

- Avoid the sun.

- Follow the antiaging program outlined in the next chapter.

- Use a moisturizer.

- Use an exfoliant if you need it. See the information on alpha hydroxy acids (AHA) later in this chapter.

# blackheads

Most teenagers—and some adults—are all too familiar with blackheads. Blackheads are not caused by dirt; they are formed by an extrusion of an oily substance from the glands and debris from discarded cells from the inside of a hair follicle. This causes a plug that can become either a whitehead or, as the surface dries out, a blackhead. To get rid of it:

- Use salicylic or glycolic acid pads.

- Wash your face gently with sand grains. If you don't live near the beach, you can use a homemade oatmeal scrub.

- Use face-blotting paper. Cut the paper into little pieces and blot the skin every few hours to absorb extra oil.

# crow's-feet

Crow's-feet are usually associated with middle age, but can occur in people in their twenties, particularly if they have light-colored eyes, are nearsighted, and squint. Professional treatments are discussed in the section on cosmetic treatments. In the meantime, here are some tips to help prevent squinting, a major cause of crow's-feet:

- Wear sunglasses.

- Wear a hat or visor in the sun.

- Make sure your glasses, contacts, or sunglasses are the correct prescription.

- Use a moisturizer and sunblock daily around your eyes.

# dry scalp

Our scalp is always being abused. Because our hair is the focus of much of our vanity, we subject our scalp to hair sprays, the heat from blow dryers, coloring chemicals, and more, all to mold our hair into the latest style. We pay for these abuses, most commonly with a dry irritated scalp and hair that over time becomes frayed and damaged. Aside from stopping all of the abuse (which we're not asking you to do), here are some tips to keep your hair healthy. But remember, if your scalp gets very dry and flaky, make an appointment with a dermatologist.

- Don't wash your hair every day if you don't need to, especially if your hair is short. Shampoos, no matter how gentle, are very drying, and hair rarely gets so dirty as to require detergent washing. For that healthy bounce, though, condition your hair every day to replenish the moisture and provide some protection from the abuse that is likely in the offing.

- Don't wear your hair in a ponytail or braid it. This can damage your hair and result in what is referred to as "traction alopecia," or a thinning of the hair. This particularly occurs at a woman's hairline from the constant tightness of wearing the hair pulled back.

- Get the tips of your hair trimmed frequently to minimize split ends. As with any crack or fray, once a split starts it can easily progress.

- Set your blow dryer on the cooler setting when drying your hair. This minimizes heat damage both to the hair and to the cuticle, its protective layer. You can turn the heat up to style it.

- Occasionally use an overnight conditioner, such as a peanut oil–based product. Rub it through your hair and cover your hair with a shower cap overnight.

## dry skin

As we age, our skin becomes drier. If you were plagued with pimples as a teenager, chances are that's not your problem now. So you need to take action to restore that facial dew. Dry skin is more often a problem in winter or when the seasons change. The important things to remember are to moisturize and not dry out your skin. Here are some tips:

- Take short showers or baths.

- Take warm—not hot—showers and baths. Breaking the hot-water habit is one of the best things you can do to maintain the moisture balance of your skin.

- If possible, decrease bathing in winter to every other day.

- Use soap to wash only under your arms and your groin area.

- Add bath oil, not bath salt or bubbles, to your bathwater.

- Use Crisco moisturizing cream. This is our favorite low-cost, homemade potion. You can use it after every bath or shower. Use it alone or alternate it with a cream that contains alpha hydroxy acid. Just dissolve 2 tablespoons of salt in 2 cups of hot water, then mix in a blender with 1 pound of Crisco. Apply the cream to your damp skin immediately following your bath or shower.

# irritated skin

These are soothing remedies if your skin is irritated from a new makeup or if you're having an allergic reaction to a spray or other chemical.

- Make a milk compress. Simply mix equal parts of whole milk and ice water. Soak a handkerchief or wad of tissues in it and apply it to the irritation. Because milk is a base, not an acid, this is very soothing. Use this compress for ten minutes four times daily, decreasing the amount of time each day.

- Take an aspirin or a nonsteroid antiinflammatory, such as ibuprofen or Aleve, to decrease the inflammation.

- Make a green tea compress. Soak a green tea bag in water, let it set until room temperature, dip tissues into the tea, and apply.

- Apply a compress made with ice water to the irritation.

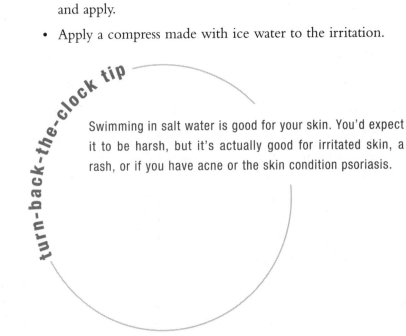

turn-back-the-clock tip

Swimming in salt water is good for your skin. You'd expect it to be harsh, but it's actually good for irritated skin, a rash, or if you have acne or the skin condition psoriasis.

# lip lines

Vertical lip lines are one of the first signs of aging. They can be inherited and/or caused by sun damage. They are particularly annoying because lipstick makes them appear more prominent. Permanent solutions are outlined in chapter 7. Meanwhile, to help prevent them:

- Don't smoke.

- Don't whistle.

- Don't pucker up. (Okay, maybe we're going too far with that one . . . forget it!)

- Use moisturizer and sunblock around your mouth.

- Use lip liner.

- Use Vaseline, Aquaphor, or other lip balm morning and night to keep your lips supple and smooth.

# pimples or acne cysts

You're all dressed to go out, and suddenly a pimple or acne cyst erupts. This was bad enough as a teenager, but now you're not supposed to suffer such indignities. You could get a cortisone shot from your doctor to help deflate the pimple immediately, but the office is closed. Try these remedies:

- Apply a dab of benzoyl peroxide.

- Apply a dab of strong cortisone cream.

- Apply a dab of toothpaste and leave it on overnight.

## sweating

Excessive sweating causes both physical and social discomfort. Sweating can be embarrassing, ruin clothing, make you feel insecure, and interfere with social and business interactions. There are ways to treat excess underarm and foot sweating, such as BOTOX injections. But before doing that, though, try a deodorant that contains aluminum chloride.

## swelling around the eyes

This is by far the most common complaint we hear. Puffy eyes make people look tired and older than their years. As you age, fat is extruded from the orbit of your eye, creating this puffy look. This puffiness is more obvious when the fat cells swell with water, which is exactly what occurs when you lie flat or ingest salt. Laser eyelid surgery, or blepharoplasty (see chapter 9) is the permanent solution. Here are some temporary measures:

- Sleep on two or three pillows.
- Place books underneath the top part of your bed to raise it.
- Decrease your salt intake.
- Rest with a cold compress over your eyes. Try an ice mask, a bag of frozen peas, cucumber slices, cold spoons, or gauze soaked with water.

# thinning skin
# (resulting in black-and-blue marks)

Not all black-and-blue spots come from trauma. As you grow older, your skin thins and becomes fragile. Buy arnica cream in your local health food and vitamin store and apply it twice daily. We often use this cream to speed healing after procedures that cause bruising.

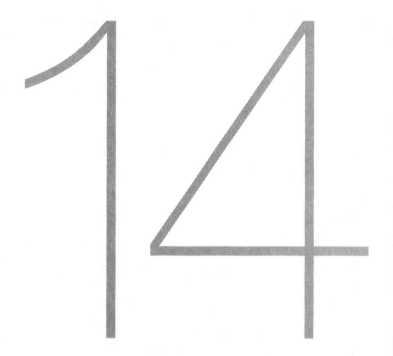

# 14

## PREVENTION: HOW TO

## SLOW DOWN THE CLOCK

The most important thing you can do to maintain a youthful glow is to follow a program of prevention. By caring for your skin diligently with a good skin-care regimen, you'll look better. You can start such a program at any age—if you're young, this program will help you stay looking that way longer. And if you're older, your skin will look its best.

We're often asked if people need to see a dermatologist to be put on a sound skin-care regimen. If you're younger, with normal skin, following a program like this may very well be all you need. If you have skin problems, such as severe acne, eczema, or psoriasis, you should consult a dermatologist. Whether you're older and concerned about your aging skin, or younger but your skin has suffered a lot of sun damage, a single consultation with a cosmetic dermatologist can put you on the right track.

In this section, we'll mention the types of products that you can find at the drugstore or cosmetic counter that can help you maximize your skin's health.

No matter which products you choose, begin by using a "trial and error" approach. If you haven't been using a program, it's tempting to jump in, buy everything you need, and start using it immediately. Don't do that! Buy one product at a time and try it alone for a few days. Pay attention to how your skin reacts. What is good for one person is not always good for another. If your skin becomes irritated, then stop, wait a few days, and try another brand of the same type of product. If the product seems fine for your skin, repeat the procedure with the next product, and so on. For instance, if you try a glycolic acid gel, and your skin pores gradually become smaller, it's working. But if you get a rash or irritation with any product—stop using it.

It's best to follow a program created by a dermatologist, not the "consultant" at the cosmetics counter of your local department store. Sometimes major brand cosmetics are great, but cosmetic consultants are salespeople, and you might end up with more than you need. You also may be given erroneous information and/or inflated claims. For years we've been dealing with an epidemic of acne where we didn't expect to see it: among women in their midtwenties. Paula, twenty-five, had the slightly oily skin you would expect in a woman her age. She told the saleswoman at her local cosmetics counter that she wanted to begin a skin-care program. She was sold a cleanser, a toner, and a moisturizer. The toner did remove the oil from her skin—in fact, it removed too much. The moisturizer was designed to replace this lost oil. The result was that she developed acne. She would have been better off retaining some of that natural oil rather than artificially replacing it. The resulting acne is very common in such cases: we refer to this as "acne cosmetica"—cosmetic-caused acne.

Some oil in your skin isn't necessarily bad. Most people have a certain amount of their natural oil, which helps keep them from getting wrinkled and dry. You don't want to have greasy skin, but on the other hand, you don't want to dry it out, either, because your natural oil is the best for your skin. It holds in moisture and keeps your skin feeling smooth and supple.

When it comes to buying cosmetic products, don't chose creams solely because of the vitamins they contain. A good moisturizer containing vitamins can be helpful, but much of the benefit is due to the moisturizer. There is no way to determine if light has rendered them inactive by the time you buy the cream, or even whether the vitamins ever were active or whether they are effective when applied topically in a cream base. Bottom line? Although the future prospects of treating the damage of the sun's UV radiation with antioxidants such as vitamins A, C, E, and K are enticing, the creams available now probably don't live up to their billing.

# our antiaging skin-care program

## who needs an antiaging program?

Everyone. We're not just talking about women. Years ago, male cosmetic patients were rare. Today, one-quarter of our patients are men, and the number is climbing. No matter whether you're male or female, it's only natural to want to look as young as you feel.

# when should i start?

Throw away the calendar. Caring for your skin does not depend on how old you are; it depends on the condition of your skin. For instance, Debbie is a thirty-three-year-old, blue-eyed, blond, fair-skinned sun worshiper whose dry, damaged skin is starting to wrinkle. Carla, thirty-five, with brown eyes and an olive complexion, has skin in better condition. Both women can benefit from this program, and even though Debbie is younger, she will need a heavier moisturizer. That's an example of how this program can be customized to suit the particular needs of your skin. Generally, beginning this antiaging program at about age thirty-five is ideal, but if you are very fair skinned, or have suffered sun damage, you may need to start earlier.

## antiaging facial morning treatment

1. Wash your face with a gentle cleanser.

2. Apply a glycolic acid–based gel and let it dry.

3. Apply sunscreen or sunblock to your entire face.

4. Apply a moisturizer if your skin is dry.

5. Apply makeup if desired.

The first step is to use a very mild nonsoap cleanser. The facial cleanser you use should also be hypoallergenic. A good one, Cetaphil, is widely available at drugstores. Others are Aquanil Lotion and Liquid Neutrogena Facial Formula.

Our "no soap" edict may surprise you, but we are serious about it. Soap is drying. We'll never forget one of our patients who came to see us. She had just turned thirty, yet her skin was so severely wrinkled she seemed a candidate for a face-lift and facial resurfacing. It turned out that the culprit was the soap she was using on her face. This facial bar was almost 100 percent pure detergent soap, and it dried out her skin's natural oils. After a week of following our skin-care program, her skin was smoother and unlined again. This is an extreme example, but it demonstrates the importance of proper skin care.

After cleansing your skin, apply a glycolic-based acid gel. This is a mild exfoliate, which will provide a gentle skin peel. Experiment with strengths to find the one that works best for you.

Glycolic gel is made with glycolic acid, which is an alpha hydroxy acid (AHA), made from chemicals found in a variety of fruits. Research finds that products that contain AHA acids can product modest antiaging effects. AHA products cause exfoliation, or the shedding of dead cells from your skin's epidermis. AHAs are made from a variety of fruit, including apples, grapes, or citrus fruits. The exfoliation effects of AHA can make your skin look brighter and feel smoother. The AHA concentrations found in over-the-counter products are generally about 10 percent; products with higher concentrations are used in chemical peels. If your AHA product stings or irritates your skin, consider using a product that doesn't have AHA. Also, since AHA exfoliates dead skin cells, this will make your skin more sun sensitive, so don't forget to put on your sunscreen next.

No matter what your age, and no matter what season it is or what the weather outside is, apply a sunscreen or sunblock product. Any broad-spectrum (UVA and UVB ray) protector of at least 15 SPF is fine. There is no evidence a higher number than that is more effective. Then, especially if you're going to be out in the sun, you can add an extra layer of sun protection and reapply with prolonged exposure.

Do you need a moisturizer? Let your skin type be your guide. If your skin is oily, don't use it; if your skin is not oily, do.

Moisturizers come in different weights—gels (the lightest), lotions (light), and creams (heavier). Use the right one for your skin. If you need just a little moisturizing, pick a gel. If you need a medium amount, use a lotion, and if your skin is very dry, use a cream.

When you use a moisturizer, pat some water on your face first. The water will hydrate your skin and the moisturizer you apply will lock in the extra hydration.

## antiaging night facial treatment

If you're young (in your teens to your early twenties), you only need to cleanse your face at night, as you did in the morning. If your skin is dry and sun damaged, also use a moisturizer. If you're older, you'll want to use Retin-A or a similar product to guard against wrinkles. Here's the nighttime program:

1. Cleanse your face with the gentle cleanser.

2. On alternate nights, apply Retin-A or a similar product to your entire face, excluding the upper eyelids over the globe of the eye. Then, five to ten minutes later, apply a moisturizer, followed by a moisturizing eye cream.

3. On the days you don't use Retin-A, use the moisturizer and a moisturizing eye cream.

If your skin is very dry, you may want to skip using a cleanser and just gently clean your face with water. Never use a washcloth on your face. It's too rough. If you're older, with dry skin, use a gentle exfoliate to slough off the dead skin cells.

## retin-a

Tretinoin—the active ingredient in Retin-A, Renova, and Retin-A Micro—is the only FDA-approved medication proven to improve the appearance of sun-damaged skin. These products are available only by prescription. If you're serious about preventing wrinkles, consider seeing a doctor and getting a prescription. The over-the-counter substitute, retinol, doesn't have quite the level of effectiveness, but many women find it's all they need.

If you are using Retin-A, retinol, or a similar preparation, and you are planning to be in the sun a lot, stop using it for three days beforehand. Also, stop using it three days before waxing the area and one week before electrolysis or laser hair removal.

# our antiaging skin-care program for men

You'll want to ward off premature aging as well. You can easily protect your skin by following a simple skin-care program like the one outlined for women—but even simpler. When you're young, just use a mild cleanser. As you get older, you might want to add glycolic acid gel in the morning, followed by a sunscreen or sunblock. If you have a bald spot, don't forget to put sun protector on it! At night, use the cleanser and Retin-A or retinol, on alternate days, as prescribed above. If softer skin is what you seek, you can use glycolic gel at night.

Follow these steps and, no matter what your age, your skin will look the best it can.

# taming the sun: your skin's greatest threat

When it comes to taking care of your skin, there are two main rules to follow. If you stick to these rules, your skin will improve.

**Rule 1. Avoid the sun.**

**Rule 2. Follow Rule 1.**

As we noted in the last chapter, 90 percent of the signs associated with aging, such as lines, wrinkles, and dark spots, actually come from sun exposure. To minimize this aging, you must minimize your time spent baking in the sun.

We know our tirade against the sun seems almost like a crime against nature. It's become a natural reaction to view someone pale as unhealthy—"You're so pale, dear; have you been sick?" Conversely, we consider someone with a bronze hue to be healthy—"You look great! You must have been on vacation!"

This wasn't always so. At the turn of the century, women paraded around the shore toting parasols. Pale skin was a sign of the upper class, while a ruddy complexion denoted the working class who toiled outdoors. Remember the Gabor sisters, Zsa Zsa, Eva, and Magda? They looked decades younger than their years for their whole lives. Their Hungarian mother had wisely shielded them from the sun since birth.

We're not referring only to the damage that comes from sunbathing; we're also referring to the damage you get when you just go about town with unprotected skin. The danger from sun radiation is not from the dozen or so times each season you go to the beach, but the radiation from the sun year-round, including winter, spring, and fall. Still, you can do real damage—like seeing coin-size brown spots emerge on your skin—from the exposure you'll get on a Caribbean island.

So what's so bad about the sun?

The sun is a giant ball of radiation. Radiation is transmitted in two different types of rays—UVA (ultraviolet A) and UVB (ultraviolet B) rays. (There's a third type—UVC—that can't radiate through the ozone layer, so we don't have to worry about that—yet.) Sun damage is cumulative over your lifetime.

Both UVA and UVB rays can cause sunburn. But there are less obvious effects as well. Although UVA rays produce less skin redness than the shorter UVB rays, they do deeper damage. These

UVA rays can travel through clouds and even reach your skin through closed glass windows. The UVA rays can also cause skin cancer, a problem of epidemic proportions.

We know it's impossible to completely avoid the sun, and we wouldn't want you to. Hey, we're in favor of a Caribbean vacation as much as anyone. We also know that you will go out in the sun simply because it feels so good. So the important rule here is: when you know you're going to be in the sun, or just outside, protect your skin. Sit under an umbrella, use a sunblock, and wear a hat, and be especially careful from 11 A.M. to 2 P.M., when the sun's rays are the strongest.

When it comes to your skin and the sun, there's the bad news and the good news. The bad news is that 80 percent of the damage from the sun to your skin is done by the time you're twenty years old—it just takes years for the signs to become obvious. Also, the fairer-skinned and lighter-eyed you are, the more important sun protection is. The good news is that it is never too late to protect yourself, even though the skin never forgets the radiation it has received.

The first thing to do is to use sunscreen. Using sunscreen also helps protect against skin cancer. Although most skin cancer is curable when caught early, it can be disfiguring.

Sunscreens are protective substances that extend the length of time you can safely stay outside. You judge the protectiveness of a sunscreen according to its SPF, which stands for its sun protection factor. For example, if your skin ordinarily turns pink after 10 minutes, a sunscreen with an SPF of 15 extends this to 2½ hours (ten minutes × the "15" protection factor equals 150 minutes).

We don't mean for you to get out a calculator every time you want to go out into the sun; the above math simply underscores the point that even if you use sunscreen, don't bake in the sun indefinitely. Let your complexion be your guide as well. If you're olive skinned, you can stay out longer than your fair-skinned counterpart.

What about tanning parlors? Stay out! The notion that getting a tan is protective before summer or going on a sunny vacation is a myth! Furthermore, tanning parlors often use more of the damaging UVA rays. No matter where your sun exposure comes from, whether from sunbathing or lying in a tanning parlor, this radiation is damaging!

## safe sunning tips

Here are some recommendations for how you can protect yourself from the sun:

- Purchase sunscreen or sunblock and get into the habit of applying sun protection as part of your everyday skin-care regimen, not only in the summer. Buy a sun-protection product of at least SPF 15. If you're fair-skinned, choose one that is SPF 30. There is no evidence higher numbered products afford significantly more protection, but it may last longer throughout the day. Make sure the sun protection product is labeled "broad spectrum," which means that both UVA (ultraviolet A) and UVB (ultraviolet B) rays are screened out.

- Apply sunscreen liberally. Put it on fifteen to twenty minutes before going out. If you're swimming or sweating, reapply often.

- Don't forget to put sunscreen on these commonly missed areas: the V of your chest, your ears, the backs of your hands, and the sides of your neck.

- If you're very fair or are going to be sunning yourself, add a physical sunblock. These are products that say they contain zinc oxide or titanium dioxide on the label. They used to be a thick substance but now are "micronized" and go on thinner.

- Limit your sun exposure between 10 A.M. and 2 P.M., when ultraviolet rays are the strongest.

- Wear a hat and a long-sleeved shirt or clothing made with fibers that screen out the sun's rays.

- Want some color without the sun damage? Experiment with the self-tanning products available from the major cosmetic companies. This new generation of products won't streak or turn you orange.

- The best way to protect your hair from sun damage is to wear a wide-brimmed hat when going outdoors. If your hair is color treated, it may be very prone to sun damage. Also, if you have bleached, frosted, or highlighted hair, and plan to take a dip in a chlorinated pool, wear a swim cap or, at the very least, use a special swimmer's shampoo and hair conditioner. This isn't as good as a cap, but they can help remove some of the chlorine so your highlights don't turn a fetching shade of green!

# skin cancer:
# what you need to know

This is a book about beauty, and there's nothing that can mar your appearance like the disfiguring surgery sometimes necessitated by skin cancer. Since you'll be paying close attention to your skin as you read this book, this is an ideal time to learn a little about skin cancer. That way, you can take note of any suspicious abnormalities you find and bring them to the attention of your dermatologist.

Why be concerned about skin cancer? Because the skin cancer rate is soaring, with about 1.3 million new cases expected this year. Melanoma, the less common but more malignant form of skin cancer, is also increasing.

There are three forms of skin cancer: squamous cell, basal cell, and melanoma, which take their names from the three layers of cells that make up our skin. Most skin cancer involves the skin's outer layers, squamous and basal cell; melanomas arise from the deeper melanin cells.

Melanoma is the deadliest form. The other two forms of skin cancer, although highly curable, can be disfiguring if left untreated for a long time. But, when diagnosed early, these forms of skin cancer can be treated with excellent results.

Risk factors for skin cancer include:

- A family medical history of skin cancer or melanoma.

- Being fair skinned and having light-color eyes.

- Prolonged sun exposure.

- Having had one or more bad sunburns in the past, especially when you were young.

## screening for skin cancer

The best screening test for skin cancer is one you do yourself. This is called a skin self-exam and involves examining your skin for abnormal growths and moles. To begin, stand naked before a full-length mirror. Examine your scalp, parting your hair into small segments. Look over your entire body. Check your genitals, the inside of your mouth, the backs of your ears and your soles. Use a small hand mirror, or ask your partner, to check your back. If you find a new mole or skin marking, or if a marking apparently has grown, changed color, or looks or feels different, contact your doctor or dermatologist. Remember, melanoma can appear anywhere, but in women it most commonly occurs on the arms, trunk, head, neck, and especially the legs.

## moles

Most of us have a number of small, colored, harmless-seeming spots on our body—moles, freckles, and birthmarks. We are usually born with a few, and the rest develop throughout our life. Most moles are normal and remain so. But some families have a lot of moles, and often the moles are very abnormal. People in some of these families are at risk for developing melanoma.

Moles also change as we age. Adolescents and young adults tend to have dark, flat moles that become slightly elevated and begin to lose color as they age. So by the age of eighty, people rarely have very dark moles. However, mole changes that do not occur as part of the normal aging process are those that should be checked. Here are some signs to pay particular attention to:

- A mole that grows larger.

- A mole that forms an irregular border.

- A mole that changes in color.

- Inflammation that forms around a mole.

part3

# Putting It All Together

We've covered the ways you can rejuvenate, maintain, and take care of your skin. We've told you about all of the current technologies and the future directions of cosmetic dermatologic surgery. But now what? All this information can be dizzying. The important question remains—how do you determine what treatment is best for you?

The cosmetic dermatological field today is one marked by choice. As we noted at the beginning of this book, years ago the choices were limited and those that existed involved invasive, risky procedures that required a lot of recovery time. Now the choices are great. Dermatological surgeons can choose or combine several techniques to solve almost any common cosmetic problem.

This section shows you the various treatments and how they are combined to solve a myriad of cosmetic problems while keeping recovery time to a minimum.

# review of problems and solutions

## problem—abdominal scars
## solution—subcision and liposuction

Abdominal scars can be separated from the underlying skin and excess tissue removed with liposuction.

## problem—acne scars, face

## solution—laser peel, subsurface tightening/toning, filling substances, punch graft

To eliminate or improve acne facial scars, a number of techniques can be used alone or in combination, depending on the extent of the scarring. Laser peels can smooth the skin, making the scars less visible. The Erbium YAG laser and the $CO_2$ laser are used for this purpose. Lasers for subsurface tightening/toning can also be used for acne scars with no down time. Soft-tissue filling substances such as collagen, Dermalogen, Restylane, silicone, or fat can be injected to elevate depressed scars. The "punch graft" technique can also be used.

## problem—acne scars, back
## solution—peels, laser subsurface toning/tightening

A medium-depth chemical peel can help eliminate or reduce the appearance of some acne scars. Cool touch or medlite laser resurfacing (toning/tightening) won't completely remove the scars, but it can make them much less noticeable. Filling substances can also be injected to elevate depressed scars on the back, just as they can be used to improve the appearance of facial acne scars. Stronger lasers cannot be used on the back.

## problem—baggy eyelids
## solution—blepharoplasty, laser resurfacing

The main way to get rid of baggy eyelids is through blepharoplasty. For the upper lid, an incision is made in the natural crease, and extra skin and fat are removed. Fat from the lower lid is removed from the inside of the lid so there is no outside scar. This is called a transconjunctival blepharoplasty. But if the problem is mild laser resurfacing can be done instead, with blepharoplasty reserved for later use. Laser resurfacing can also be used with or after blepharoplasty to enhance the results and tighten the skin.

## problem—benign growths

## solution—scalpel shaving; desiccation and curettage; electrodissection; chemical ablation; surgical excision; liquid nitrogen; laser surgery with $CO_2$, Erbium, and Pulsed-dye lasers

All of these methods refer to different ways to remove benign (noncancerous) growths. They can be shaved off, surgically removed, lightly burned off, or removed with chemicals, liquid nitrogen, or lasers.

## problem—blood vessels
## solution—Pulsed-dye laser

An overabundance of blood vessels can cause reddishness on the skin. Some people have one or two darker red areas. To get rid of this problem, we use a laser light specifically absorbed by the blood so that the vessels can be destroyed while leaving the rest of the skin unharmed.

## problem—brown spots
## solution—ND: YAG laser, Ruby laser, Alexandrite laser, chemical peels, desiccation

Some brown spots are caused by sun damage. There are various ways of removing them, depending on their size and location and your skin tone. One of the three lasers above can be used, or a chemical peel can be done to improve the appearance of the entire area. The brown spot may also be melted away with an electric machine, a process called desiccation.

## problem—hollow or sunken cheek
## solution—fat transfer

Hollow-looking cheeks convey an aged, skeletal look. Fat can be harvested from elsewhere on the body and injected into the cheeks to fill them out.

## problem—crepey skin

## solution—antiaging skin-care program plus chemical peel, or microdermabrasion with laser subsurface toning/tightening, LILAX or $CO_2$ laser resurfacing

To help prevent crepey, or aged, skin, follow our antiaging skin-care program. To firm up the skin, a chemical peel, microdermabrasion with laser toning/tightening, or laser resurfacing using the $CO_2$ laser are the solutions. If the crepelike skin is not confined just to the face but also hangs in folds on the neck, LILAX— the combination of liposuction, laser, and excision that is done under local anesthesia—may be an excellent choice.

## problem—crow's-feet

## solution—BOTOX, filling substances, fat transfer, chemical peels, laser peels, microdermabrasion with subsurface laser toning/tightening

There are many ways to deal with crow's-feet, the "squint" lines on the sides of the eyes that are among the earliest signs of aging. The treatment choice depends on how severe the lines are and what other problems you want to take care of on the face. BOTOX can erase lines; filling substances and fat transfer can fill them in; chemical, laser peels, and microdermabrasion with subsurface toning/tightening smooths them.

## problem—cysts
## solution—excision

Cysts, which are benign, sebum-filled growths on the skin, can be easily removed by cutting or simply by making a hole in the skin and "popping" the cyst out.

## problem—dark circles (under eyes)
## solution—ND: YAG or Ruby laser, $CO_2$ laser resurfacing, chemical peel, filling substances (collagen or hyaluronic acid), fat transfer, bleaching agent

Dark circles under the eyes are the result of several contributing factors, so often a combination of treatments works the best. The darkness may be caused by increased heredity pigment, fat that extrudes from the orbit of the eye, causing a shadow beneath it, or from the skin thinning out, revealing the darker underlying tissue underneath. The solution is filling substances, which can take care of the hollowed look or the thin skin. For pigmentation, bleaching sometimes works. But when it doesn't (which is often), a medium chemical peel, or laser resurfacing with the $CO_2$ or Erbium laser, can take care of the problem.

Both these lasers tighten and lighten the skin. Transconjunctival blepharoplasty, a procedure using the laser, can be performed to remove the excess fat.

## problem—double chin
## (known also as turkey neck, jowls)
## solution—liposuction, LILAX

Fat doesn't collect only on our waist and thighs. As we age, it also collects on our face and neck. Fortunately, using liposuction on the face, jowls, sides, or folds around the mouth, chin, and cheeks can easily empty these pockets of excess fat. Over the following months, the skin tightens and rests more firmly against the structure of the face. For those with significantly loose skin, the LILAX procedure (liposuction, laser, and excision) is performed with similar ease and recovery time. In this case, a small portion of the skin is removed from under the skin, and the undersurface is tightened by small incisions with a $CO_2$ laser. Areas on the face can also be treated in the same way. At the same time fat transfer is performed to enhance other areas.

## problem—earlobes

## solution—for long or ripped holes: surgical repair; for thin/elongated earlobes: filling substances (collagen, Dermalogen, hyaluronic acid, silicone), fat transfer

A pierced earlobe that is ripped through due to an earring is a common problem that can be surgically repaired. At the same time, if the hole has become too long, it can be surgically shortened. Thin, elongated, droopy earlobes, caused by aging, can also be made plumper and younger looking using filling substances or tightened using $CO_2$ laser resurfacing.

## problem—eyelids, excess skin and fat, upper lid
## solution—blepharoplasty, resurfacing

Blepharoplasty, upper eyelid surgery, with or without resurfacing, can smooth this area.

## problem—eyelids, excess fat, lower lid
## solution—transconjunctival blepharoplasty

Using a laser, the physician makes an incision inside the lower eyelid and removes the fatty deposit. The laser coagulates the blood as it cuts, preventing bleeding. This laser procedure requires no stitches and is performed under local anesthesia.

## problem—eyelids, excess skin, lower lid
## solution—laser resurfacing, subsurface tone/tightening, chemical peel or $CO_2$ laser

These solutions used to tighten skin elsewhere on the face can also be used to smooth, lighten, and tighten excess skin below the eyelid.

## problem—facial contour defects
## solution—LILAX, liposuction, filling substances

With aging, the bony and fatty structure of our face shrinks, causing our eyes and cheeks to appear hollowed. Our eyebrows sag and lose their arch. For the floppy chin area, LILAX, the combination of liposuction, laser resurfacing inside the skin, and excision, provides much of the benefit of a face-lift without having to resort to that far more extensive procedure. Facial depressions caused by this shrinkage can be rebuilt with some permanence by using filling substances and fat transfer.

## problem—fat (excess body)
## solution—liposuction

Using tumescent liposuction with local anesthesia to get rid of excess amounts of fat in trouble spots all over the body is one of the most exciting and satisfying fields within cosmetic surgery. Here's a list of the problem areas that can be treated with this procedure safely and with no or little recovery time.

### abdomen

Whether you call it a "pot," "pouch," or "tummy," the fact is that no one wants excess fat here. This is true for men and women. But for some women liposuction of the waist or abdomen can sometimes result in an unfeminine boxy form. So the Hourglass Abdomen procedure was born. This three-pronged approach applies liposuction to the abdomen, waist, back, and hips for an instantly shapelier look.

### arms and underarm bulges (bra fat)

Liposuction can firm up saggy upper arms by removing excess fat. Liposuction can also remove the excess fat that bulges in front of and behind the underarms.

## breast and chest (men)

Men sometimes develop excess fat in their chest area that can resemble female breasts. This excess fat can be removed with liposuction.

## calves and ankles

The unflattering nickname "piano legs" is often given to women with excess fat around the lower calves and ankles. Liposuction can remove this excess fat, resulting in more attractive, shapelier legs and ankles.

## dowager's neck

See **Double Chin.**

## face

See **Facial Contour Defects.**

## hips

Excess fat can be removed with liposuction from the hips. Some women just have large hips, but others have enlarged hips as part of what is known as a violin deformity. See **Thighs—Outer (and Violin Deformity).**

## waistline (women); love handles (men)

As women grow older, it's very common for excess fat deposits to make a waistline vanish. Liposuction can come to the rescue and whittle away the excess fat to recapture that sculpted look. For men, this excess fat can result in "love handles." These can also be easily removed to restore that youthful physique.

### thighs—inner

Liposuction can get rid of the excess weight that accumulates between inner thighs and causes them to uncomfortably rub together.

### thighs—outer (and violin deformity)

Known also as "saddlebags," this is the name given to excess fat that accumulates on the outer thighs. A woman can even be very thin and have fat deposits in this area. Liposuction of the upper thighs is often combined with that of the hips and buttock ("violin deformity") to achieve the best results. Liposuction can also be performed around the entire thigh to reduce the diameter of the leg.

### knees

Liposuction can remove excess fat from the inside and top of the knees, resulting in slimmer legs and a better look in skirts.

### buttocks

Some women who believe they have "saddlebags" actually have excess fat in their buttocks. In this case, liposuction alone can be used to create a far more flattering bottom.

### problem—excess hair
### solution—laser hair removal, electrolysis

Electrolysis is the permanent removal of unwanted hair by means of shortwave electric current, which destroys the hair's roots. A more modern choice, however, is laser hair removal. A number of different lasers are used to remove hair; the best for you depends on your skin type and the color of the unwanted hair. Laser hair removal is now available for most people, although there are a few exceptions, such as people with gray and extremely light blond hair. Here are the body areas that lasers can treat: for women, hair can be removed from the underarms, legs, and bikini area; for men, from the ears, hands, knuckles, back, and chest.

## problem—forehead lines
## solution—BOTOX, filling substances, $CO_2$ laser resurfacing, subsurface toning/tightening

There are a number of ways to treat forehead lines. BOTOX can be used to selectively relax muscles, erasing lines. Filling substances and fat transfer can also be injected to soften lines and make them less visible, while lasers are used to smooth and tighten the skin.

## problem—frown line
## solution—BOTOX, filling substances, $CO_2$ laser

The frown line, which is the vertical line between the eyebrows, is one of the problems people are eager to treat because it not only makes them look older but it also makes them look angry. In most cases, BOTOX can be used to erase the line, but for more deeply etched lines, filling substances may be needed to make this prominent line less noticeable, and lasers can help smooth the area.

## problem—jowls

see **Double Chin.**

## problem—turkey neck

see **Double Chin.**

## problem—hair loss

## solution—hair loss medications: finasteride (Propecia), spironolactone, and minoxidil (Rogaine); hair transplant, scalp injections

This problem occurs in both men and women. In men, hair loss can begin as early as their twenties and result in baldness. In women, hair loss usually begins after menopause and manifests itself as thinning hair, rather than baldness. If the problem is in its early stages, and not that much hair has been lost, medications may be sufficient. Rogaine (minoxidil) comes in two strengths, one for men and one for women. Rogaine is not that effective; it usually takes about four months for any growth to be noticed, and the Rogaine must be used indefinitely. Because of its drawbacks, Rogaine is sometimes more effective when used as a supplement with another method, such as the oral medication Propecia (finasteride). This medication can offer dramatic results to men. Older women find mixed results. Women of childbearing years cannot take Propecia, but they can take spironolactone with good results. Scalp injections with a low-dose steroid can sometimes help halt hair loss.

Both men and women benefit from hair restoration surgery. For men, the modern method of transplanting hair involves taking hair from the back of the head, which never stops growing, and transplanting it to the balding areas. For women, grafts are taken from the growing hair in back and grafted between the existing hair follicles, to give a fuller appearance. Newer methods of using micrografts and minigrafts create an even more natural effect. Men with extensive baldness may need more than a hair transplant; they may require scalp reduction, which involves reducing the area of the bald scalp by surgical excision, then pulling upward and lifting the hair-bearing skin together. This decreases the size of the bald patch.

## problem—hollows (under eyes)
## solution—$CO_2$ laser, chemical peel, subsurface toning/tightening, filling substances (collagen, Dermalogen, Restylane, silicone), fat transfer

See **Dark Circles (under eyes).**

## problem—hollow cheeks
## solution—fat transfer

Hollow cheeks can be plumped up by the restoration of some of the natural substances in our skin, which decrease as we age. Fat implants can restore a pleasing fullness to the cheeks.

## problem—lipoma
## solution—excision, liposuction

These benign growths of fatty tissue, which commonly occur on the forearms, torso, or the back of the neck, can be easily taken care of by making a small incision and removing them. If there is a large lipoma, this can be removed with liposuction combined with excision.

## problem—lips, thin

## solution—filling substances (collagen, Dermalogen, Restylane, silicone), fat transfer

Young, plump lips are one of the most aesthetically pleasing parts of the body. But with age, the tissues shrink, and this thins the lips. Fortunately, the lips are easy to inflate. Almost any of the filling substances can be successfully used here. Collagen traditionally has been used. Since it doesn't last that long, though, other substances may be preferable. Your physician can select which substance is best for you.

## problem—lip lines (vertical)

## solution—$CO_2$ laser resurfacing, subsurface tightening/toning, dermabrasion, filling substances (Zyderm I and II, Restylane); for fine lines: hyaluronic acid, BOTOX.

Vertical lip lines are usually one of the earliest signs of aging and are particularly distressing because lipstick makes them appear more prominent. $CO_2$ laser resurfacing, subsurface tightening/toning and filling substances, BOTOX, or a combination of two or more of these solutions can help solve this problem.

## problem—marionette (puppet) lines

## solution—filling substances (collagen, Dermalogen, hyaluronic acid, silicone, BOTOX), fat transfer

Marionette lines, those depressions that start from the corner of the mouth and sag downward toward the chin, are best treated with different types of filler. Often, fat transfer is used to build up the area; then the superficial wrinkle and the sagging corner of the lip can be enhanced and raised with collagen or hyaluronic acid.

## problem—moles
## solution—scalpel shaving, excision

Most moles are harmless and, if unsightly, can be easily removed in a physician's office. A tiny amount of local anesthetic is injected and the mole (or nevus) is shaved off flush with the surrounding skin. This permanently removes the mole 98 percent of the time. In the rare cases the mole recurs, it can be excised, or cut away again. If hair grows out of the mole, that can be removed by electrolysis, a device that uses electrical current.

## problem—nasolabial lines
## solution—filling substances (collagen, hyaluronic acid, silicone, Dermalogen), fat transfer

Nasolabial lines, the common "smile" lines between the nose and the mouth, can be filled in with filling substances. Collagen or hyaluronic acid (Restylane), silicone, or Dermalogen are the most common. If the lines are deep, the person's own fat, Gore-Tex, or silicone are excellent choices. These substances fill in more deeply and last longer.

**problem—nevi**

**solution—See *moles*.**

**problem—neck sagging**

**solution—liposuction, LILAX**

Excess fat can be removed from a sagging neck by the use of liposuction alone, or combined with laser resurfacing and excision in a procedure known as LILAX. For this process, liposuction is performed to remove fat around the neck; laser resurfacing under the skin tightens it and a small piece of skin under the chin is excised in its natural crease so the loose skin can be lifted a bit. The result is not as dramatic as a face-lift but provides great improvement using local anesthesia and a far shorter recovery time.

**problem—red/rosy skin**

**solution—Pulsed-dye laser (V-Beam)**

A variety of different types of red, rosy skin and red spots are caused by abnormally dense or dilated blood vessels showing through the skin. This can result in a variety of problems that includes spider angiomas (bright red areas with slender projections resembling spider legs), port-wine stain (flat, pink, red, or purple discoloration appearing at birth), telangiectasia (enlarged vessels), cherry hemangiomas (those cherry red bumps people get with age), and rosacea (a chronic skin condition). Usually the Pulsed-dye V-Beam laser can destroy these blood vessels, leaving the rest of the skin undamaged.

**problem—rosacea**

solution—see *red/rosy skin*

**problem—puppet lines**

solution—see *marionette (puppet) lines*

**problem—sallow skin**

solution—antiaging skin-care program, chemical peels, microdermabrasion, laser resurfacing ($CO_2$ laser, Erbium laser), subsurface laser toning/tightening

As we age, our skin gets more dull and sallow; chemical peels and resurfacing brighten it.

**problem—scars**

solution—see *acne scars*

**problem—traumatic and other scars**

solution—Pulsed-dye laser, $CO_2$ laser, laser toning/tightening, and excision

Using lasers to resurface is a modern way to remove scars; laser tightening/toning can also help smooth the area. Some scars can also be shaved with a scalpel. Cortisone injections can also make scars less raised and noticeable.

**problem—skeletal hands**

solution—fat transfer, sclerotherapy

The loss of tissue that comes with aging can make hands look skeletal. Fat transplants can plump them up, and sclerotherapy, a method that destroys protruding veins, can restore their youthful smoothness.

## problem—sun damage
## solution—antiaging skin-care program, sun protection, chemical peels, microdermabrasion, $CO_2$ laser, Erbium laser, subsurface laser toning/tightening

Sun damage causes wrinkles, red spots, brown spots, and sagging. The best treatment for sun damage is prevention by using sunscreen daily, year-round. Many treatments also can help reverse the damage. To make a difference requiring very little recovery time, there are a variety of options, including laser toning, microdermabrasion, and light chemical peels. Treatments that offer more significant results are medium-depth chemical peels and Erbium laser resurfacing or $CO_2$ laser resurfacing.

## problem—sunken cheeks
## solution—fat transfer

As we grow older, the structure of our face changes, and once-rounded cheeks can appear sunken. An injection of your own fat is the best way to restore their pleasing plumpness.

## problem—sweating, excessive
## solution—Botox, liposuction, and excision

Botox can be used for excessive sweating that occurs under the arms, on the palms, or on the feet. Multiple injections right under the skin in the desired areas after topical anesthesia stun the sweat glands for six months at a time. Another option for underarm sweating is liposuction, which is performed very superficially under the skin to scrape out the sweat glands. Since sweating usually occurs in a small area (the underarm), excising a piece of skin that has the sweat glands that sweat the most is performed.

### problem—tattoo removal
### solution—Alexandrite, ND: YAG, Ruby, and Pulsed-dye lasers

Lasers have made tattoo removal much easier, but it still remains a difficult task. Different lasers must be used depending on the color ink used. Given the elaborateness of today's designs and array of colors, tattoo removal can take many treatments. Success also varies according to the skin and ink colors: the easiest to remove are dark colors on light skin. But even given these problems, tattoos can be successfully removed, or at least made far less noticeable.

### problem—"turkey neck"
### solution—(see *double chin*)

### problem—varicose and spider veins
### solution—sclerotherapy, ambulatory phlebectomy, lasers

Sclerotherapy is the best and most common treatment for spider veins. It involves injecting the veins with a mild irritating solution that irritates the vein walls and causes the vessels to be absorbed by the body. For more pronounced varicose veins, ambulatory phlebectomy is used. This involves using local anesthesia to numb the area, making a series of pinpricks along the vein and teasing it out.

# resources

RHODA S. NARINS, M.D.
DERMATOLOGY SURGERY & LASER
CENTER
1049 Fifth Avenue
New York, NY 10028
212-288-9910

DERMATOLOGY SURGERY & LASER
CENTER
222 Westchester Avenue
White Plains, NY 10604
914-684-1000
http://narins.com

DR. PAUL JARROD FRANK
FIFTH AVENUE DERMATOLOGY
SURGERY & LASER CENTER
1049 Fifth Avenue, Suite 2B
New York, NY 10028
212-327-2919

Drs. Narins and Frank offer a line
of skin-care products used in their
practices. For more information,
go to www.narins.com,
www.pfrankmd.com, or www.
turnbacktheclockwithoutlosingtime.com.

AMERICAN SOCIETY FOR
DERMATOLOGIC SURGERY
930 E. Woodfield Road
Schaumburg, IL 60173-4927
847-330-9830
1-800-441-ASDS (2737)
http://www.asds-net.org

AMERICAN ACADEMY OF
COSMETIC SURGERY
Cosmetic Surgery Information
Service
737 N. Michigan Avenue
Suite 820
Chicago, IL 60611
312-981-6760
http://www.cosmeticsurgery.org

AMERICAN ACADEMY OF
DERMATOLOGY
P.O. Box 4014
Schaumburg, IL 60168-4014
847-330-0230
www.aad.org

INTERNATIONAL SOCIETY FOR
DERMATOLOGIC SURGERY
930 N. Meacham Road
Schaumburg, IL 60173
847-330-9830, extension 373

# Index

# about the authors

Dr. Rhoda Narins is a clinical professor of dermatology at New York University Medical Center, where she teaches advanced dermatologic cosmetic surgery and heads the liposuction surgery unit. She is the director of the Dermatology Surgery and Laser Center in Manhattan and Westchester. She is a diplomate of the American Board of Dermatology, a fellow of the American Academy of Dermatology (AAD), a member and former member of the Board of Directors of both the American Society for Dermatologic Surgery (ASDS) and the International Society for Dermatologic Surgery (ISDS), and a fellow of the American Academy of Cosmetic Surgery (AACS). In addition, Dr. Narins is the Chief Emeritus and a senior attending in the department of dermatology at White Plains Hospital Medical Center.

Dr. Narins, an innovator in the field of liposuction cosmetic surgery, lasers, and fat transfers, lectures and teaches throughout the world on these and other cosmetic procedures. She has published textbooks on cosmetic surgery and safe liposuction and has written numerous articles pertaining to cosmetic surgery. Dr. Narins has been named in "the Best Doctors in New York" by *New York* magazine and has been listed in *Town and Country* as one of the leading U.S. cosmetic surgeons and in "Best Doctors in America."

Dermatologic surgeon Dr. Paul Jarrod Frank is the founder and director of the Fifth Avenue Dermatology Surgery and Laser Center in Manhattan. He is a clinical instructor and director for the Cosmetic Dermatology Clinic for training physicians at New

York University Medical Center and is an attending dermatologist at White Plains Hospital. Noted for his expertise in minimally invasive cosmetic surgery, Dr. Frank has lectured extensively and authored articles and chapters pertaining to cosmetic surgery in both the professional and consumer literature. Additionally, he is regularly featured in several beauty and fashion magazines as a skin expert. Academically, Dr. Frank continues his ongoing research in dermatologic surgery, investigating new products and techniques for both the private and corporate sectors.

Dr. Frank is a diplomate of the American Board of Dermatology and is a fellow of both the American Academy of Dermatology and the American Society of Dermatologic Surgery. He trained in Internal Medicine at New York's Columbia Presbyterian Medical Center and completed his dermatology residency at New York University Medical Center.